You Are Not Sick You Are Thirsty

WATER CURES: DRUGS KILL

HOW WATER CURED INCURABLE DISEASES

F. Batmanghelidj M.D.

Author of Best Seller
Your Body's Many Cries for Water
and
Water: For Health, For Healing, For Life

GHS
Global Health Solutions, Inc.
www.watercure.com

Copyright © 2003 Fereydoon Batmanghelidj, M.D.

ISBN 0-9702458-1-5

First Edition: November 2003

Global Health Solutions, Inc., 8472-A Tyco Road, Vienna, VA 22182
Telephone: 703-848-2333
Fax: 703-848-0028
Website: *www.watercure.com*

Library of Congress Control Number 2003110089

Cover Design: Jonathan Jones
Book Design: Jonathan Jones

First Printing August 2003

To our **Creator:**

In awe, with humility, dedication, and love.

I thank the Almighty for His light and the fine-detailed guidance that has made this presentation in His name possible. At last, He has shed light on our past deep-rooted ignorance, in the name of advanced medical science, in the twentieth century.

In memory of my mother Lila: She taught me the moral values of truth, honesty, integrity, and empathy as a child.

"In the arts of life man invents nothing; but
in the arts of death he outdoes Nature herself,
and produces by chemistry and machinery all the slaughter
of plague, pestilence and famine."

George Bernard Shaw

The tragedy is in the way these killings are all legitimized, without a second thought, if any profit can be made from such immoral deeds.

The *Washington Post*, Wednesday, April 15, 1998: Correctly Prescribed
Drugs Take Heavy Toll: *Millions Affected by Toxic Reactions*;
by Rick Weiss, *Washington Post* staff writer,
highlights the very theme of this book:

The Washington Post

WEDNESDAY, APRIL 15, 1998

Correctly Prescribed Drugs Take Heavy Toll

Millions Affected By Toxic Reactions

By RICK WEISS
Washington Post Staff Writer

More than 2 million Americans become seriously ill every year because of toxic reactions to correctly prescribed medicines taken properly, and 106,000 die from those reactions, a new study concludes. That surprisingly high number makes drug side effects at least the sixth, and perhaps even the fourth, most common cause of death in this country.

You now have proof that prescription drugs do really kill: read the rest of the book to discover how easily water has cured serious diseases, and why.

Author's Note

The information and recommendations on water intake presented in this book are based on training, personal experience, very extensive research, and other publications of the author on the topic of water metabolism of the body. The author and producer of this book does not dispense medical advice or prescribe the use or the discontinuance of any medication as a form of treatment without the advice of an attending physician, either directly or indirectly. The intent of the author, based on the most recent knowledge of microanatomy and molecular physiology, is to offer information on the importance of water to well-being, and to help inform the public and medical professionals of the damaging effects of chronic unintentional dehydration on the body, from childhood to old age.

This book is not intended as a replacement for sound medical advice from a physician. On the contrary, sharing of the information contained in this book with the attending physician is highly desirable. Application of the information and recommendations described herein are undertaken at the individual's own risk. The adoption of the information should be in strict compliance with the instructions given herein. Very sick persons with a past history of major diseases and who are under professional supervision, particularly those with severe renal disease, should not make use of the information contained herein without the supervision of their attending physician.

This book is intended to open your eyes to new possibilities that would ultimately emancipate societies throughout the world from the dark age of medicine that has become established on the foundations of scientific ignorance of the human body, and the fraud of those who preserve the status quo and make money in the process. You are urged to read more on the topic before you begin to apply the information to your own personal health problems. This request is intended to protect you against jumping to conclusions, without recognizing the ramifications of possibilities within your reach.

All the recommendations and procedures herein contained are made without guarantee on the part of the author or the publisher, their agents, or employees. The author and publisher disclaim all liability in connection with the use of the information presented herein.

CONTENTS

Introduction

There is a medical breakthrough that is not reaching the public through our medical schools or health-maintenance organizations: the discovery that *chronic unintentional dehydration* is the primary cause of pain and disease in the human body, including cancer. The reason these traditionally trusted institutions do not celebrate this scientific discovery and refuse to use it to help the sick and the uninsured poor in our society is obvious. There would be no money in it for them.

What we in medicine did not realize until very recently is the fact that the human body can become short of water inside its cells even when water is available, plentiful, and virtually free. Imagine, more than one hundred years of serious scientific research has been conducted on the solid composition of the body–obviously and totally oblivious to the vast complications that ensue when the body is dehydrated; when its plum-like and juicy cells become transformed into prune-like and drying cells because of insufficient water, or due to the additionally dehydrating beverages that are on the market now.

When the gradually dehydrating body begins to malfunction and manifest its water shortage, we label these symptoms and signs of the body's regional and local drought as diseases or syndromes of unknown origin (diseases of unknown etiology). And since the discovery of DNA structure, we now blame genes for a patient's health problems—obviously not realizing that when any cell begins to dry up and get damaged from inside, the nucleus in that cell, and its DNA structure, are not exempt from the process.

Twenty-two years of my full-time research has brought about the medical breakthrough that I am now sharing with you. Initially I tried to get the medical community to process my information and incorporate it into their treatment protocols. My sincere enthusiasm and hope proved to stem from my naïveté. What I was proposing—to treat dehydration of the body with water and not toxic medications that do more damage to the patient than they do good—was not complicated enough to impress the patient and glorify the doctor; nor would this new treatment approach perpetuate the sickness and make money for the doctor over a longer period of time. Naturally, if patients were to know that their health problems were caused by not drinking enough water, why would they go to the doctor's office again? For this reason, institutional doctors did not acknowledge this medical breakthrough. They gave it the silent treatment and forced me to take my information directly to the public.

Society has to be warned about the present (2003 AD) ignorant understanding of the human body's symptoms of persistent drought in the interior of its cell. This "inside-the-cell" regional water shortage is not reflected in current investigative procedures, which measure the solid components of the circulating blood. Blood formation is designed in such a way that its composition is standardized, even if other tissues have to sacrifice some of their reserves to achieve this. Water is one of these elements that will be taken away from less active areas and used to maintain the consistency of blood, if sufficient amounts do not become available from external sources of supply—that is, from drinking.

When the gradually dehydrating cells in drought-stricken areas of the body become inefficient and produce symptoms that denote water shortage, modern medicine, instead of using brain power to identify the *physiologic* reasons for the *"dis-eases"* that ensue from water shortage, has called these same conditions *diseases* and has designed treatment protocols that depend on the use of killer chemicals. Suffering from drought is bad enough, but then they go and further burden the body with toxic chemicals in the name of advanced medical science.

Naturally, making money is the primary incentive here. The money-making approach to dis-eases of dehydration in the past century has financed the growth of the "sick-care" system, which survives and thrives from people staying dehydrated but "symptom-free"; they use chemicals that silence the many cries of the body for water. This is the reason society is burdened with monumental sick-care costs that grow 12 percent every year—I am told that the total figure is now around $1.7 trillion and rising.

The insurance companies are constantly raising their rates; at the same time, they methodically trim their coverage, shifting the burden of expenses more and more onto their clients. No wonder we now have more than forty million people who are uninsured in America—the land of plenty, also the land of shameless self-serving exaggerations. I am sure you remember the media reports on all those CEOs whose companies were failing—and yet they paid themselves tens of millions of dollars, year in, year out, as their companies went belly-up.

The sick-care system is no exception, except that the public had to make the sacrifice and pay whatever they asked, every time. We needn't buy a car that is too expensive, but no matter the unreasonableness, we have been forced to pay the exorbitant rates demanded for health services. The good news I am sharing with you is the scientific fact that the thoroughly researched health information in a glass of water is going to turn this trend and its actors on their heads. Within the next few years most of these establishments are going to realize that the public will no longer be fooled by medical theatrics and jargon-protected treatment protocols. One by one, people will discover water as a primary medication for most of their health problems.

Do you know what is going to happen? When this book, with all its medical reports, and my other books and educational materials, eventually reach the hands of "ambulance-chasing" lawyers, then people who have lost children to asthma or other serious complications of dehydration and who received toxic and harmful medication when all their bodies needed was water will take their doctors and their institutions to court for having done them harm. The drug companies will be sued for planting misinformation in medical schools for financial gain. When this information hits the fan, the National Institutes of Health, the FDA, the drug companies, even the medical schools and their medical journals, as well as the fund-raising medical foundations, will run to the nearest body of water to cleanse themselves from the stench of involvement in their ignorant and fraud-driven crimes against humanity. Strong words, but that is exactly how I see it. Why do I see it this way?

The report of my having successfully treated with simple tap water more than three thousand persons with symptoms and clinical signs of peptic ulcer disease was published in the *Journal of Clinical Gastroenterology* in June 1983. I came away from that experience with the understanding that the people I treated were all thirsty, and I uncovered the phenomenon that "pain" in the body indicates thirst, even though the condition is classified as a disease.

The *Science Watch* of the *New York Times* made an announcement about this event, and the article was syndicated and published in quite a number of other newspapers. Twenty years have passed since then, and we are still treating heartburn with strong antihistamine medications or antacids. Why? Because there is no money in prescribing water for a patient who is in pain. Water would cure the pain produced by dehydration, but medications convert the patient into a "cash cow" for the sick-care system. Am I too cynical? Not in the least. I am offended by the way medical ignorance has been fostered and closely protected by the pharmaceutical industry, with the thoughtless and unwitting partnership of the mainstream medical community, all of it at the expense of the trusting public. Why do I think in this way?

I set out to scientifically prove my discovery about pain as a marker of water shortage in the body. I asked myself why the pharmaceutical industry insisted on treating peptic ulcer disease with very strong antihistamine medication. What is the relationship of histamine to pain? These were the questions I started to research.

I went to the library of the University of Pennsylvania in Philadelphia, where I was extended the privileges of a visiting scholar by Professor Michael (Mitch) Litt, then chairman of the Bioengineering Department; one of his fields of interest was the structure of mucus. When he found out about my research on pain and water, he suddenly realized the rationale behind the structure of mucus. It consists of 2 percent solid scaffolding and 98 percent water, which is trapped and held within the meshes of the scaffolding. He realized that the biological purpose behind the design of mucus is to serve as a moist layer that protects exposed-to-air membranes from becoming dried up. Until then all mucus specialists were concentrating on the 2 percent solid matter in mucus and oblivious to the reason for entrapment of water within the structure.

Initially I spent four years, sometimes eighteen hours a day, reading medical articles, scientific articles, proceedings of various conferences on brain messenger chemicals (neurotransmitters), and books published within the discipline of biophysics to understand the "relationship of water to life." I was sure my answers could only be found in the latter publications and not in the medical journals. I was right.

I discovered a very serious error in the medical understanding of the human body. It is not solid matter that regulates all functions of the body; instead, it is water that dissolves all the solid matter it circulates in the blood and *provides energy* for chemical reactions in *all of the functions* of the body. In short, water is the master regulator; everything else is subservient. Instinctively, we knew that, but those in medicine were told otherwise.

The foundation of our medical knowledge has been based on a number of false assumptions about water. This is the reason we have a sick-care system and not a disease-preventing health-care system. Such a system can only come into being through scientific research within the discipline of physiology, and not the jargon-peddling application of toxic and death-forwarding chemicals to the human body. Just take a look at the list of warnings about any one of the drugs that are pushed on television or in print advertising.

In September 1987 I gave the opening address of an international cancer conference in Greece. In this lecture I explained why pain is one of many cries of the body for water; and why it is chronic unintentional dehydration that is the primary cause of pain and disease in the human body, including cancer. My article "Pain: A Need for Paradigm Change" was published by the *Journal of Anticancer Research* in their September–October issue. I was asked to give the lecture after a peer-reviewed evaluation of the scientific reasons for my proposed paradigm shift by the then head of the Tumor Biology Unit of King's College Medical School of London University. A conference was convened to expose this new information to other cancer researchers. The *Journal of Anticancer Research* is a prestigious and well-read journal in the field of cancer research.

The Scientific Secretariat of the 3rd Interscience World Conference on Inflammation, having come across my findings that histamine is a neurotransmitter in charge of water regulation and drought management of the body and its role in pain production, which denotes thirst, invited me to expand on this view in their conference in 1989 in Monte Carlo. The abstract of my presentation follows, allowing you to see why water is a better natural antihistamine than anything the pharmaceutical industry offers.

3rd INTERSCIENCE WORLD CONFERENCE ON

INFLAMMATION
ANTIRHEUMATICS, ANALGESICS,
IMMUNOMODULATORS.

ABSTRACT FORM

IMPORTANT: These instructions must be followed completely.
Read all instructions before you begin typing on this special
form.

Mail to
Scientific Secretariat
3rd Interscience
World Conference
on Inflammation
Istituto di Farmacologia
Via Roma, 55
56100 Pisa (Italy)

Title

Authors

Institute

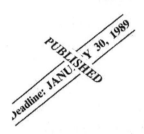

FORMAT FOR ABSTRACT

1. Your abstract should be infor-
mative, containing: (a) specific ob-
jectives; (b) methods; (c) summary
of results; (d) conclusions.
2. Single space all typing. Capitalize
all letters of the title. The text
should be a single paragraph, starting with a 3-space indentation.
Leave no top or left margin within
the area provided.
3. Abbreviations must be spelled out
on first mention, followed by the
abbreviation in parentheses.
4. Any special symbol that is not on
your typewriter must be drawn in
BLACK INK.
5. DO NOT ERASE. Remember that
your abstract will appear in a
special volume exactly as sub-
mitted.
6. Mail first class with 2 photocopies
to address given above.
7. If more than one abstract is sub-
mitted with the same first author,
indicate which abstract should
have priority. Other abstracts will
have a lower priority.
8. **Please underline speaker's name.**

NEUROTRANSMITTER HISTAMINE :
AN ALTERNATIVE VIEW POINT

F. Batmanghelidj, M.D.

Foundation For The Simple In Medicine,

ABSTRACT: Advances in histamine research show it to be a neurotransmitter, a
neuromodulator and an osmoregulator of the body. While thirst sensation is a failing indicator
of now recognized, age-dependent, state of possible cellular and chronic dehydration of the
body, to the point that between the ages of twenty to seventy the ratio of the extracellular to the
intracellular water content of the body has been shown to change from a figure of 0.8 to almost 1.1, histamine is demonstrating responsibility for the essential osmoregulatory and
central dipsogenic functions in the body. Histamine is involved in the initiation of cellular
cation exchange, that seems to be supplemental to the role of water in cellular metabolic
mechanisms. Histamine is also a modulator of lymphocyte biology and function; through H_1
or H_2 activation of the different lymphocyte subpopulations that have nonrandom distribution of histamine receptors, their functions are integrated. Histaminergic drive for body water
regulation and intake brings about the release of vasopressin, which in turn, by possible
production of "shower head" cluster perforations of 2 Angstrom units, allowing single file
entry of one water molecule at a time through the membrane, promotes increased flow of water
through the cell membrane; this function is particularly important for the maintenance of the
low viscosity, microtubule directed, microstream flow of the axonal transport system. Vasopressin seem also to act as a modulating cortisone release factor, when constant ACTH secretion can
be implicated in the general inhibition of the immune system's functions; histamine may be
involved in modulation of neuroendocrine systems, possibly when ACTH feedback
mechanism is broken. Next to oxygen water is the single most essential substance for the
survival of the body, also recognizing that the dry mouth is not the sole indicator of "free water"
deficiency of the body, symptom producing excess histaminergic activity, including chronic
pain production, should be judged to be also an indicator of body water metabolism imbalance. The natural primary physiological drives of the histaminergic, the serotonergic
neurotransmission (another system involved in the body water regulation, as well as pain
threshold alteration) and the angiotensin II for water intake of the body should be acknow-
ledged and satisfied before and during evaluation of the clinical application of antihistamines
in treatment procedures, particularly as increased water intake may be the only natural process
for the regulation and inhibition of histamine's over production and release. The prolonged
use of antihistamines in gastroenterological, psychiatric, seasonal allergic conditions, as analgesics or anti-inflammatory agents without very strict attention to body water intake
regulatory functions of histamine, by also masking signals of dehydration, may eventually
be the cause of cell membrane receptor down-regulation and disturb the integration and
balance, and possibly, shift the immune system in an opposite dominant direction and therefore, be responsible for the production of new and continuing change of physiological
steady-state situations, incompatible with the total and prolonged well-being of the patient.

Key Words: *Histamine, pain, inflammation, immunomodulation, thirst, water*

PUBLISHED; PAGE 37 OF THE ABSTRACT VOL.
3rd Interscience World Conference On Inflammation,
Antirheumatics, Analgesics,Immunomodulators.
Monte-Carlo (Principality Of Monaco), March 15-18, 1989
In Win 89

If we look at histamine within its role as a water regulator of the body, the entire structure of medicine will change and become people-friendly, and the science of physiology will take over. At present, the medical industry fraudulently and knowingly presents histamine as a nuisance substance and produces chemical substances that interfere with and block its actions. All drugs used as pain medications, as anti-allergy medications, as antidepressants and tranquilizers are directly and indirectly very strong antihistamines. And yet water is an infinitely better natural antihistamine than all of them. They cannot do enough research on histamine to produce their drugs without understanding the natural functions of histamine in the body. The pharmaceutical industry does not possess a single drug that can compete with water as a natural antihistamine. All its drugs have serious side effects; water has none. At the same time, it performs its functions—which the different actions of histamine were trying to temporarily mimic until more water could get into the system.

You now see why I am a world-recognized professional in my field of research. My findings will force future medical research to be performed through the discipline of physiology. It will be understood that all health problems will have to be viewed as "deficiency disorders," with water on top of the list of the elements that need to be evaluated. When it is understood what element is deficient, and thus causing the health problem, its simple correction is all that would be needed. We are lucky that all the elements the body needs are incorporated within the structure of different naturally available food substances. This is why you should look at food with the idea that it is ultimately your medication and will ensure your better health, provided you become selective in what you eat.

Double-blind randomized trials *are only suited* for evaluation of *toxic chemicals* and are *not* suited for research of deficiency disorders. Such methodology of research is an obstruction to research within the discipline of physiology or nutrition. My proposed approach will produce a better understanding of how various disease conditions can be prevented. Obviously all dehydration-produced disease can be cured naturally without hurting people. The medical community has no right to hurt people by prescribing toxic chemicals to treat thirst in the body. Making a few more bucks from people's pain and suffering just because they have limited knowledge about the importance of water to their health is not an honorable way to live.

To obstruct the spread of information about water by presenting the double-blind stumbling block as is even more dishonorable. You cannot double blind the study of water as a natural medication. What are you going to compare it with? In any case, dehydration manifests itself not by a single symptom or sign, but by a number of concurrently occurring problems that the availability of water will reverse. When you read the letters that are presented in this book, you will understand what I am saying. In no way can you apply the drug industry's methodology of research to evaluation of water as a "natural medication." Any sugges-tion to the contrary would only delay the emergence of water as a most effective natural medication, to the chagrin of the public and elation of the drug companies. They could continue to terrorize the public into using their products for a while longer by more media advertising.

To show you some insight into my ongoing battle with the medical establishment, which insists on staying in the dark ages of medical sci-ence when a simple change of focus could catapult the entire system of medical education to the highest orbit of possibilities in understanding the human body, I have chosen to include three samples of my efforts. One is an e-mail letter to an upcoming star of Harvard University. Another is an article of mine on thirst that was published in January 2003 issue of *Townsend Letters for Doctors and Patients*. The third article is on the terrorism of the drug industry; it has been posted on my Internet site for the past year. What surprises me is the fact that I am still alive to continue.

I sent my article on thirst as an attachment to the e-mail letter to the Harvard doctor.

To: www.osher-institute@hms.harvard.edu

Sent: Saturday, November 30, 2002 5:31 PM

Subject: Re: Newsweek Article — The Science of Alternative
Medicine/Dr. Eisenberg   Sat 11/30/02

Dear Dr. Eisenberg:

"A new scientific truth is not usually presented in a way to convince its oppo-nents. Rather, they die off, and a rising generation is familiarized with the truth from the start." **Max Planck**

I read the *Newsweek* article with much interest. I noticed that you were well projected in all that was written, as if the whole piece was about you. Obviously you are also a very active member of the medical community that is interested in steering medicine away from its enslavement to the pharmaceutical industry. If this is the case, I would like to introduce you to an entirely new physiology-based approach to the etiology of pain and disease in the human body.

Twenty-two years ago I started treating peptic ulcer disease with water. In two years and seven months, I had successfully treated over 3000 cases. I came away from that experience with the understanding that these people were really thirsty: That we in medicine had labeled one of the manifestations of thirst in the human body as a disease condition (particularly as a number of other conditions also responded to increased water intake).

My report of the treatment process was published as the editorial of the *Journal of Clinical Gastroenterology* in June of 1983. I then set out to prove why these people were only thirsty. In September of 1987 I presented the guest lecture of an international cancer conference under the title of "Pain: A Need for Paradigm Change" and declared the *"solutes-regulatory"* paradigm obsolete. I explained that it is the *"solvent"* that regulates all the physiological functions of the body. I explained that it is *"chronic unintentional dehydration"* that is the etiology of pain and the degenerative diseases, including cancer: That all these conditions are the result of *"system disturbance"* because of the missing action of water. To prove my point of view, I had shown that histamine is actually a neurotransmitter in charge of water regulation and the drought management programs of the body. My presentation is published in Sept.–Oct. issue of the *Anticancer Research Journal* in 1987.

In 1989, the Scientific Secretariat of the 3rd Interscience World Conference on Inflammation, etc. invited me to make my presentation of histamine at their conference. The abstract of my presentation "Neurotransmitter Histamine: An Alternative View Point" is attached. [Note: In this book it appears on page 7.] These, and many other articles on the topic of the *"molecular physiology/pathology of dehydration,"* are posted on my website *www.watercure.com*.

Not only the primary cause of pain and the degenerative diseases of the human body seem to have emerged from my research, the uncanny simplicity of their prevention has also become clear—prevent dehydration to prevent disease!!

To show you how stagnant medical thinking at prestigious medical schools is, and how it is hurting the public, I have taken the liberty of adding my rebuttal letter to Dr. Valtin of Dartmouth College, School of Medicine to this letter.

My dear Dr. Eisenberg, if you ponder the way the water industry has grown in the past 10 years, you will realize that my information, presented in my books, newspaper and magazine articles, in addition to many thousands of radio interviews, has already impacted the public's desire to stay healthy. Some secondary schools are teaching my books. In California they passed a resolution to throw soda-vending machines out of the schools. The rising new generation of Americans is becoming acquainted with the information on preventing thirst. If medical schools, such as Harvard, wish to remain as significant as they are, they need to engage in the research of the *"solvent"* paradigm. You are so beautifully situated to engage in this topic; it would be a crime to let the opportunity pass you by. I know you are impressed by Chinese medicine, but tell me, if people learn to prevent pain by drinking water, how many would go to an acupuncturist for the hell of it?

If you go to my website and wish to have some of my educational products to share with others in your office, please let me know, I will send them to you as a gift.

Sincerely, F. Batmanghelidj, M.D.

Waiting to Get Thirsty Is to Die Prematurely and Very Painfully

F. Batmanghelidj, M.D.

Author: *Your Body's Many Cries for Water*

Heinz Valtin, M.D., an emeritus professor at Dartmouth Medical School, has ventured the opinion that there is no scientific merit in drinking 8 x 8-ounce glasses of water a day and not waiting to get thirsty before correcting dehydration. This view, published in the *American Journal of Physiology*, August 2002, is the very foundation of all that is wrong with modern medicine, which is costing this nation $1.7 trillion a year, rising at the rate of 12 percent every year. Dr. Valtin's view is as absurd as waiting for the final stages of a killer infection before giving the patient the appropriate antibiotics. His views are based on the erroneous assumption that dry mouth is an accurate sign of dehydration.

Like the colleagues he says he has consulted, Dr. Valtin does not seem to be aware of an important paradigm shift in medicine. All past views in medicine were based on the wrong assumption that it is the solutes in the body that regulate all functions, and that the solvent has no direct role in any of the body's physiological functions. In medical schools it is taught that water is only a solvent, a packing material and a means of transport; that water has no metabolic function of its own. I have come across this level of ignorance about the primary physiological role of water at another Ivy League medical school from another eminent professor of physiology who, like Dr. Valtin, researched and taught the water-regulatory mechanisms of the kidney to medical students and doctors. Only when I asked him what "hydrolysis" is did the penny drop: He admitted the scientific fact that water is a nutrient and does indeed possess a dominant metabolic role in all physiological functions of the body.

Dr. Valtin's emphasis on the water-regulatory role of the kidneys limits his knowledge to the body's mechanisms of "deficit management" of the water needs of the body. He seems to base his views of thirst management of the body on the vital roles of vasopressin, the antidiuretic hormone, and the rennin-angiotensin system, the elements that become engaged in the drought-management programs of the body, when the body has already become dehydrated. Indeed, he thinks dehydration is a state of the body when it loses 5 percent of its water content; and that one should wait until at some level of such water loss the urge to drink some kind of "fluid" will correct the water deficit in the body. This view might have seemed plausible 25 years ago. Today, it exposes the tragic limitations of knowledge of the human physiology that is available to a prestigious medical school in America.

In his recently published and widely reported assertions, Dr. Valtin does not take into consideration the fact that water is a nutrient. Its vital "hydrolytic" role would be lost to all the physiological functions that would be affected by its shortage in its osmotically "free state." Another oversight is the fact that it is the interior of the cells of the body that would become drastically dehydrated. In dehydration, 66 percent of the water loss is from the interior of the cells, 26 percent of the loss is from extracellular fluid volume, and only 8 percent of the loss is borne by the blood tissue in the vascular system, which constricts within its network of capillaries and maintains the integrity of the circulation system.

Philippa M. Wiggin has shown that the mechanism that controls or brings about the effective function of the cation pumps utilizes the energy-transforming property of water, the solvent: "The source of energy for cation transport or ATP synthesis lies in increases in chemical potentials with increasing hydration of small cations and polyphosphate anions in the highly structured interfacial aqueous phase of the two phosphorylated intermediates[1]". Waiting to get thirsty, when the body fluids become concentrated before thirst is induced, one loses the energy-generating properties of water in the dehydrated cells of the body. This is a major reason we should prevent dehydration, rather than wait to correct it. This new understanding of the role of water in cation exchange is enough justification to let the body engage in prudent surplus water management rather than forcing it into drought and deficit water management, what Dr. Valtin is recommending that people do.

In his research on the "conformational change in biological macromolecules," Ephraim Katchalski-Katzir of the Weizmann Institute of Science has shown that the "proteins and enzymes of the body function more efficiently in solutions of lower viscosity[2]". Thus, water loss from the interior of the cells would adversely affect their efficiency of function. This finding alone negates Dr. Valtin's view that we should let dehydration get established before drinking water. Since it is desirable that all cells of the body should function efficiently within their physiological roles, it would be more prudent to optimally hydrate the body rather than wait for the drought-management programs of the body to induce thirst. Furthermore, it is much easier for the body to deal with a slight surplus of water than to suffer from its shortfall and have to ration and allocate water to vital organs at the expense of less vital functions of the body. The outcome of constantly circulating concentrated blood in the vascular system is truly an invitation to catastrophe.

The tragedy of waiting to get thirsty hits home when it is realized that the sharpness of thirst perception is gradually lost as we get older. Phillips and associates have shown that after 24 hours of water deprivation, the elderly still do not recognize they are thirsty: "The important finding is that despite their obvious physiologic need, the elderly subjects were not markedly thirsty[3]". Bruce and associates have shown that, between the ages of 20 to 70, the ratio of water inside the cells to the amount of water outside the cells drastically changes from 1.1 to 0.8.[4] Undoubtedly this marked change in the intracellular water balance would not take place if the osmotic push and pull of life could favor water diffusion through the cell membranes everywhere in the body—at the rate of 10^{-3} centimeters per second. Only by relying on the reverse osmotic process of expanding the extracellular water content of the body, so as to filter and inject "load-free" water into vital cells by the actions of vasopressin and the renin-angiotensin-aldosterone systems—when the body physiology is constantly forced to rely on its drought-management programs—could such a drastic change in the water balance of the body result.

Two other scientific discoveries are disregarded when Dr. Valtin recommends people should wait until they get thirsty before they drink water. One, the initiation of the thirst mechanisms is not triggered by vasopressin and the renin-angiotensin systems—these systems are only involved in water conservation and forced hydration of the cells. Thirst is initiated when the Na^+- K^+-ATPase pump is inadequately hydrated. It is water that generates voltage gradient by adequately hydrating the pump proteins in the neurotransmission systems of the body[1]. This is the reason the brain tissue is 85 percent water[5] and cannot endure the level of "thirst-inducing" dehydration that is considered safe in the article published by Dr. Valtin.

Two, the missing piece of the scientific puzzle in the water-regulatory mechanisms of the body, which has been exposed since 1987, and Dr. Valtin and his colleagues need to know about it, is the coupled activity of the neurotransmitter histamine to the efficiency of the cation exchange; its role in the initiation of the drought-management programs; and its role in the catabolic processes when the body is becoming more and more dehydrated[5]. Based on the primary water-regulatory functions of histamine, and the active role of water in all physiologic and metabolic functions of the body—as the hydrolytic initiator of all solute functions—the symptoms of thirst are those produced by excess histamine activity and its subordinate mechanisms that get engaged in the drought-management programs of the body. They include asthma, allergies, and the major pains of the body, such as heartburn, colitis pain, rheumatoid joint pain, back pain, migraine headaches, fibromyalgic pains, and even anginal pain[5,6]. And since vasopressin and the renin-angiotensin-aldosterone activity in the body are subordinates to the activation of histamine, their role in raising the blood pressure is a part of the drought-management programs of the body[6]. Their purpose of forced delivery of water into vital cells demands a greater injection pressure to counteract the direction of osmotic pull of water from inside the cells of the body, when it is dehydrated.

From the new perspective of my 22 years of clinical and scientific research into molecular physiology of dehydration, and the peer-reviewed introduction of a paradigm shift in medical science recognizing histamine as a neurotransmitter in charge of the water regulation of the body, I can safely say the 60 million Americans with hypertension, the 110 million with chronic pains, the 15 million with diabetes, the 17 million with asthma, the 50 million with allergies, and more, all did exactly as Dr. Valtin recommends. They all waited to get thirsty. Had they realized water is a natural antihistamine[5,7,8], and a more effective diuretic, these people would have been saved the agony of their health problems.

References:

• 1. Wiggins PM; A Mechanism of ATP-Driven Cation Pumps; PP-266-269, Biophysics of Water, Eds. Felix Franks and Sheila F. Mathis, John Wiley and Sons, Ltd. 1982.
• 2. Ephraim Katchalski-Katzir; Conformational Changes In Biological Macromolecules; Biorheology, 21, pp. 57-74, 1984.
• 3. Phillips PA; Rolls BJ; Ledingham JGG; Forsling ML; Morton JJ; Crowe MJ; and Wollner L; Reduced Thirst After Water Deprivation In Healthy Elderly Men; The New England Journal of Medicine, pp. 753-759, Vol. 311, No. 12, Sept. 20, 1985.
• 4. Bruce A; Anderson M; Arvidsson B; and Isacksson B; Body Composition, Predictions of Normal Body Potassium, Body Water and Body Fat in Adults on the Basis of Body Height, Body Weight and Age; Scand. J. Clin. Lab. Invest, 40, pp. 461-473, 1980.
• 5. Batmanghelidj F. M.D. Pain: A Need For Paradigm Change; Anticancer Research, Vol. 7, No. 5 B, pp. 971-990, Sept.- Oct.1987; full article posted on www.watercure.com.
• 6. Batmanghelidj F. M.D. Your Body's Many Cries for Water; Global Health Solutions, Inc.
• 7. Batmanghelidj F. M.D.; Neurotransmitter Histamine: An Alternative View; page 37 of the Book of Abstracts; The 3rd Interscience World Conference on Inflammation, Analgesics and Immunomodulators, 1989 Monte Carlo. The abstract and the full article are posted on the Web site *www.watercure.com*.
• 8. Batmanghelidj F. M.D.; *ABC of Asthma, Allergies, and Lupus*; Global Health Solutions, Inc.

Needless to say, after I received an acknowledgment from a member of his staff that the e-mail was forwarded to Dr. Eisenberg, I did not receive any comment from the good doctor. He gave me the silent treatment, like all the others who get stunned by the gravity of what is ahead. I know how they feel. All of a sudden they feel naked. They see their many years of learning and memorization of "scientific jargons," all the statistical analysis for justification of their treatment protocols using toxic chemicals or invasive procedures, and the price structure attached to these acquired skills is declared obsolete. They realize that all they had built will soon get swept away, like a fierce slowly creeping hurricane that will reach their highly decorated home very soon. It is the public that will do it with a lot of ill feelings for the harm we in medicine have done.

Hand in hand, the drug industry has established a medical trend in America that is an infinitely more deadly form of terrorism than the kind we went to war against to avert more disasters like 9-11, not realizing that we lose more people every year to the pharmaceutical companies' brand of terrorism. The difference is in the way pharmaceutical terrorism makes money for a lot of people at the expense of a vast number of people who lose their resources before they die painfully and prematurely. I have posted the text that follows on the Internet at *www.watercure.com*. In fact, I compiled this book to expose and high-light the drug industry's brand of chemical terrorism and the media's lack of interest in what is happening. They know about the water cure and yet they have kept silent all this time.

Read my article and judge for yourself what is going on:
Where is the FDA? Where is the NIH, or the Justice
Department? Why do the very institutions designed to pro-
tect them forsake the American people?

Wake Up, America! Discover Another Deadly Form of Chemical Terrorism from Within

You Can Become Their Next Target

2002 is the year America will further expose and deal with terrorism. Americans have become aware of what havoc malice can cause for innocent and unsuspecting people—it can kill thousands with one blow. And they are not going to stand for it any longer—at any cost!

2002 will be the year Americans will realize terrorism does not solely apply to hijacking airplanes, or contaminating the postal system with anthrax spores. They will begin to appreciate that sophisticated scams against the American public that would be detrimental to the well being of the masses is yet another type of terrorism.

It is ironic that during 2002 more people will die from poor medical treatment than will die in terrorist attacks. 2001 was no different. Even though thousands of innocent people died on September 11, *many hundreds of thousands* died from wrongly administered medical treatment advice and procedures during the year 2001. Why? Why do so many people suffer and die needlessly? Why don't we see this story analyzed and reported in the media? Because we have accepted the pain and suffering of people as a norm in our society! We think pain and disease are integral parts of living. We have been brainwashed to accept this medical limitation of view about the human body and its sufferings. However, the design of the human body is not so imperfect as we have been led to believe. Surely there must be a simple natural process in the workings of the body when it is youthful, pain-free, disease-free, and in fact vibrantly healthy and joyfully alive! Surely after so many years of medical research and billions of dollars of expenditure, these natural secrets could have been found and shared with the American people. It is not as if we were short of funds and advanced technology!

The tragedy is that we have all the know-how to achieve this goal, if this were what the medical institutions wanted. The greater tragedy is that these institutions are there to make money when people are sick. Naturally, these institutions are not going to do anything that would put themselves out of business. Mournful tragedy is in the fact that the more that people helplessly abandon themselves, their health, and their savings to these "sickness-maintaining systems," the more they become brazenly greedy. It is my view that the entire system is based on an entrenched form of terrorism from within. It has established itself slowly and methodically. It operates on fear tactics and forces people into submission to get on board the doomsday train of protracted pharmaceutical death.

This situation has arisen because of a fraudulent presentation of medical science. We now know exactly how the fraud came into being. You will be fully briefed in this letter. The new scientific revelation that has been maliciously withheld from the American people to establish the medical fear tactics is as follows:

*"He is arguing for a new scientific approach that turns
clinical medicine on its head."*
The Daily Telegraph, London, England

As you can see, from the above review of my work—one of many—I am internationally recognized for my scientific research and medical background. If I were not in a very strong scientific position, I would not be able to expose the drug industry before the court of public opinion here. I am doing this for the greater good of America and the American people, who have become the victims of the worst kind of cruel terrorism known to date.

Within the discipline of physiology, the neurotransmitter histamine—a chemical the brain makes—is recognized for its primary role as a water regulator and drought-management controller. Its natural role is to coordinate physiological functions, including increased water intake until the body is fully hydrated, when its production decreases. Naturally, the more dehydrated the body, the more engaged the histamine-regulated systems become.

The process involves certain clinical manifestations that denote thirst, but have received disease labels. We might become short of breath, our joints may ache, or our blood pressure might climb, we may have more sugar in our blood, our cholesterol levels might climb, we may develop allergies, we might get splitting headaches, we might get depressed and anxious, or even develop angina, heartburn, back pain, colitis pain—and much more—all caused by shortage of water in the troubled areas. And all are treated with various drugs that function as antihistamines. This is where medicine went wrong in the first place.

Because we have, all this time, confused various symptoms of thirst with this or that disease. Because we have ignored our bodies' absolute need for water. Instead we drink junk. Caffeinated, carbonated, alcoholic, and dietary beverages have replaced water for too many of us too much of the time. And our bodies suffer the consequences, manifesting their life-threatening thirst in many different bizarre ways.

At first glance, you might think there is no relationship between thirst and all of the conditions I mentioned. But trust me, there is a most eloquent and beautiful scientific logic behind the way water shortage in the body manifests itself in all these ways—the very ways the medical community viewed as various diseases at the turn of the century, these became the themes of education in the medical schools.

The drug industry has taken advantage of this medical blind spot and has hijacked further medical education and the research priorities of the nation. It has brainwashed modern medical doctors into treating people's different natural crisis calls for water with medications. Now all physiological manifestations, or adaptive processes of the body, when it is suffering deep dehydration, are treated with this, that, or even a cocktail of chemicals. The nation has spent trillions of dollars, and about one hundred years of lost opportunity, only to kill more and more people to suit the will of a greedy few.

Thus, by the year 2001 American people have become slave workers and pay with their lives and savings to perpetuate this constantly expanding drug industry scam. The system operates on fear tactics and forces people to get on board the doomsday train of protracted pharmaceutical death. There is some outcome similarity between this functional doomsday train and Hitler's actual death trains. How else can you explain what is happening, when the body keeps crying for water and it is given toxic chemicals day after day until the person dies? As far as I can judge, and try to explain as a conscientious medical doctor, this process is nothing less than terrorism for commercial gains.

What the drug industry is doing constitutes a despicable form of terrorism against the American people. And it has to stop! The revolving doors between the FDA, the National Institutes of Health (the NIH)—its partners in crime—and the drug industry must also be replaced with concrete partitions.

Until the government steps in and stops this scam and terrorism against Americans, my friend, you had better watch out for your own self. You need to educate yourself about the ways your body speaks to you about its needs. Learn its language and make friends with it for your journey through life together. You cannot expect your body to respond normally when you give it wrong ingredients for its well-being. You cannot expect your average doctor to help you. Most doctors' past medical education, and the drug industry's aggressive sales force, did not program them with your advantage in mind. For the text of the full article on the drug industry, you might wish to visit my Web site, *www.watercure.com*.

As you saw in the *Washington Post* article, "More than 2 million Americans become seriously ill *every year* because of toxic reactions to correctly prescribed medicines taken properly, and 106,000 die from those reactions, a new study concludes. That surprisingly high number makes drug side effects at least the sixth, and perhaps even the fourth, most common cause of death in this country.

"The analysis, the largest and most complete of its kind, suggests that one in 15 hospital patients in the United States can expect to suffer from serious reaction to prescription or over-the-counter medicines, and about 5 percent of these will die as a result.

"If the findings are accurate, then the number of people dying each year from drug side effects may be exceeded only by the number of people dying from heart disease, cancer, and strokes, and may be greater than the number dying from lung disease, pneumonia or diabetes.

"Experts said the study, which appears in today's issue of the *Journal of the American Medical Association*, is stronger than previous ones because it looks only on cases in which drugs were taken correctly."

The *Washington Post*, May 7, 2002, revealed yet another drug industry trick: "Against Depression, a Sugar Pill Is Hard to Beat: Placebo Improves Mood, Changes Brain Chemistry in Majority of Trials of Antidepressants," by Shamkar Vedantam, *Washington Post* staff writer:

"After thousand of studies, hundreds of millions of prescriptions and tens of billions of dollars in sales, two things are certain about pills that treat depression: Antidepressants like Prozac, Paxil and Zoloft work. And so do sugar pills.

"A new analysis has found that in majority of trials conducted by drug companies in recent decades, sugar pills have done as well as—or better then—antidepressants. Companies have had to conduct numerous trials to get two that show a positive result, which is the Food and Drug Administration's minimum for approval."

The article is extensive and reports on research that showed placebos to be at least 5 percent more effective than the drugs under investigation. Since I have shown that the positive result of placebos may belong to the effect of water that is used to swallow a pill, and since if you get access to water, you may consume more than might be needed to wash the pill down, the antidepressant action of the sugar pill becomes less surprising than it might seem.

A brief list of conditions that are consequences of water shortage in the human body follows. When you take a look at the list, you will begin to boil like me. Why have we wasted so many years of medical research on such a gross misunderstanding of the phenomenon of thirst in the human body? Why have we hurt generation after generation of people because we were duped by the drug industry to use its toxic chemicals in place of water that the body needed to perform its natural functions? Are we responsible for making the human body more vulnerable to establishment of the degenerative disease by our jargon-peddling misinformation? Obviously, what is done cannot be reversed. Let us hope we possess enough sense and courage to correct the problem without resisting the change that is bound to take place.

Dehydration Dis-eases and Diseases

Persistent unintentional dehydration leaves its damaging impact in the fourth dimension of time. Caught in time, these conditions can be reversible, as you will read in the letters that follow.

The human body manifests it water shortage by four categories of conditions: *perceptive feelings; drought-management programs; crisis calls; and complication of persistent dehydration.*

Perceptive feelings of water shortage include: *tiredness* that is not the result of strenuous effort, such as feeling first thing in the morning that you do not wish to get out of the bed. *Anxiety, agitation, shortness of temper, depression, sleep disorders, cravings for sodas, alcohol, and even hard drugs* and *agoraphobia* are some of the ways the brain reflects its water-conservation and water-regulation problems.

The *drought-* and *resource-management* programs are: *constipation, allergies, asthma, hypertension, type 2 diabetes*, and the *autoimmune diseases.*

Crisis calls: The newly understood regional thirst signals are: *heartburn, rheumatoid joint pain, back pain, migraine headache, colitis pain, fibromyalgic pains,* and *anginal pain.*

Complications of dehydration are very extensive and include: obesity, hemorrhoids, cholesterol plaques and arterial diseases, and type 1 diabetes, as well as serious neurological disorders such as Alzheimer's disease, Parkinson's disease, multiple sclerosis, neuritis, phlebitis, lymphomas, cancers, and many more.

Medicine has traditionally divided the human body into so many specialties and subspecialties based on the different body organs' way of revealing their water shortages. Each of these groups has its own rituals for investigation within its "fiefdom." The pharmaceutical industry has accommodated physicians and has designed medications that are used in that particular "domain" of medicine. This is why, when dehydration manifests itself in more than one organ or domain of the body, the patient is forced to see many different specialists to address his or her organ-specific symptoms. Hence the use of so many different pills and treatment procedures, in the same person, for the same underlying cause—dehydration. I hope this book will shed some light on this era of medical blindness. The patient reports published in this book demonstrate how water alone naturally reverses multiple health concerns. Some of these conditions are mentioned below to help you understand the reports that follow.

Heartburn

Dis-ease: Heartburn is a signal of water shortage in the upper part of the gastrointestinal tract. It is a major thirst signal of the human body. The use of antacids or tablet medications in the treatment of this pain does not correct dehydration, and the body continues to suffer as a result of its water shortage.

Diseases: Not recognizing heartburn as a sign of dehydration and treating it with antacids and pill medications will, in time, produce inflammation of the esophagus, stomach, and duodenum, hiatal hernia, ulceration, constipation, hemorrhoids, diverticulitis, Crohn's disease, and eventually cancers in the gastrointestinal tract, including the liver and pancreas.

Rheumatoid Joint Pain

Dis-ease: Rheumatoid joint pain—arthritis—is a signal of water shortage in the painful joint. It can affect the young as well as the old. The use of painkillers does not cure the problem, but exposes the person to further damage from the medications. Intake of water and small amounts of salt will cure this problem.

Low Back Pain

Dis-ease: Low back pain and ankylosing arthritis of the spine are signs of water shortage in the spinal column and discs—the water cushions that support the weight of the body. These conditions should be treated with increased water intake—not a commercial treatment, but a very effective one.

Disease: Not recognizing arthritis and low back pain as signs of dehydration in the joint cavities of the body and treating them as different diseases with painkillers, manipulation, acupuncture, and eventually surgery will, in time, produce osteoarthritis when the cartilage cells in the joints have eventually all died. It will produce deformity of the spine. It will produce crippling deformities of the limbs. Please bear in mind: Pain medications have their own life-threatening complications.

Angina

Dis-ease: Heart pain—angina—is a sign of water shortage in the heart/lung axis. It should be treated with increased water intake until the patient is free of pain and independent of medications. Medical supervision is prudent. However, water is a natural medication for the treatment of angina.

Disease: Dehydration, to the point that it causes the heart muscles to cry for water, will produce the killer heart problems, including heart attacks, embolic problems, strokes, hypertension, heart failure, kidney disease, low oxygen distribution, edema, and more.

Migraine

Dis-ease: Migraine headache is a sign of water need by the brain and the eyes. It will totally clear up if dehydration is prevented from establishing in the body.

Disease: The type of dehydration that causes migraine might eventually cause inflammation and leakage of the small arteries of the brain and be responsible for plaque formation that is often seen in serious neurological disorders. It can also affect the back of the eye and possibly cause partial loss of eyesight.

Colitis

Dis-ease: Colitis pain is a signal of water shortage in the large gut. It is associated with constipation because the large intestine constricts to squeeze the last drop of water from the excrement—thus the lack of water lubrication.

Disease: Not recognizing colitis pain as a sign of dehydration will cause persistent constipation. Later in life, it will cause fecal impaction; it can cause diverticulitis, Crohn's disease, hemorrhoids, and polyps, and appreciably increase the possibility of developing cancer of the colon and rectum.

Asthma

Dis-ease: Asthma, which affects seventeen million children and kills several thousand of them every year, and allergies, which afflict fifty million people, are complications of dehydration in the body. Shortness of breath in asthma is a water-rationing program of the body under the control of histamine. In asthma, free passage of air is obstructed so that water does not leave the body in the form of vapor—the winter steam (we lose about one quart of water through the lungs in twenty-four hours). Increased water intake will prevent asthma attacks. It will keep every air cell better hydrated and helps them in their contraction (surface tension of water) to expel their air content every time we exhale. Asthmatics also need to take more salt to break the mucous plugs in the lungs that obstruct the free flow of air in and out of the air sacs. They also need to supplement the intake of minerals such as calcium, magnesium, potassium, zinc, and selenium, the intracellular minerals that trap water and keep it inside the cells. In dehydration, these minerals become deficient in the body.

Disease: Not recognizing asthma and allergies as indicators of dehydration in the body of a growing child not only will sentence many thousands of children to die every year, but will also permit irreversible genetic damage to get established in the remaining seventeen million asthmatic children and those who suffer from allergies. Just imagine, one-quarter of children in Harlem district of New York are reported by the *New York Times* of April 19, 2003, to be suffering from asthma. This is truly one of the great tragedies of medical ignorance and will eventually herd these innocent children onto the doomsday train of the drug industry for their shortened future lives.

Hypertension

Dis-ease: Hypertension is a state of adaptation of the body to a generalized drought, when there is not enough water to fill all the blood vessels that facilitate the normal diffusion of water into vital cells. The rise in pressure is a part of the mechanism of reverse osmosis; water from the blood serum is filtered and injected into important cells through minute holes in their membranes; extra pressure is needed for the "injection process." Just as we inject I.V. "water" in hospitals, so the body injects water into tens of trillions of cells all at the same time. Water and some salt intake will bring blood pressure back to normal! Supplements of the needed minerals to hold the injected water inside the cells would also be necessary to prevent the rise of blood pressure.

Disease: Not recognizing high blood pressure as one of the major indicators of dehydration in the human body, and treating it with diuretics that further dehydrate the body will, in time, cause blockage of the heart arteries and the arteries that go to the brain by cholesterol. It will cause heart attacks and small or massive strokes that paralyze. It will eventually cause kidney disease. It will cause brain damage and neurological disorders, such as Alzheimer's disease.

Type 2 Diabetes

Dis-ease: Adult-onset diabetes is another way the body adapts to severe dehydration. To have adequate water in circulation and for the brain's priority water needs, the release of insulin is inhibited to prevent insulin from pushing water into all body cells. In diabetes, only some cells get survival rations of water. Water and some salt will reverse adult-onset diabetes in its early stages. For full explanation on dehydration and diabetes, type 1 *and* type 2, you might want to read my book *Your Body's Many Cries for Water.*

Disease: Not recognizing adult-onset diabetes as a complication of dehydration will, in time, cause massive damage to the blood vessels all over the body. It will cause eventual loss of the toes, feet, and legs from gangrene. It will cause eye damage, even blindness. People with type 2 diabetes will eventually become insulin-dependent. They will need to receive insulin to control their blood sugar.

Cholesterol

Dis-ease: High cholesterol levels are an indicator of early drought management by the body. Cholesterol is a claylike material that is poured in the gaps of some cell membranes to safeguard them against losing their vital water content to the osmotically more powerful blood circulating in their vicinity. Cholesterol, apart from being used to manufacture nerve cell membranes and hormones, is also used as a "shield" against excessive water loss for use in other vital cells that would receive an emergency supply of water by its injection through their cell membranes. There is also a direct relationship between bones losing their calcium and getting soft and cholesterol levels, because vitamin D is made from cholesterol and exposure to sunlight. Vitamin D is needed to stimulate new bone formation. Increasing the rate of cholesterol formation might be one of the ways the body fights osteoporosis. In one of the letters, you will see how increased water intake increased bone density by 10 percent—in some bones 17 percent in the hip bone, where in encased bone density is most needed.

The classification of cholesterol as "bad" because it is seen as plaques in the arterial walls in the heart and elsewhere is inaccurate and has become a moneymaking hype for the pharmaceutical industry. We measure the body's level of cholesterol from the blood taken out of one of the arm veins. This is the blood that is moving very slowly in the veins to reach the heart. If it were the stickiness of cholesterol that caused the plaques, then the veins of the body should also get blocked; if anything, much more than in the arteries, where the blood is better mixed because of its greater pressure and the pulsating nature of blood flow. There is not a single report of cholesterol having ever blocked or formed plaques on the wall of the veins in the body. Think that one out! Actually, cholesterol serves as a "waterproofing bandage" on the abrasions and tears in the arterial walls that get damaged when the blood becomes concentrated and acidic as result of dehydration and low urine output (dark and acidic urine).

Disease: Giving cholesterol-lowering medications to people whose bodies need to make *more* cholesterol for its myriad important functions will ultimately produce many serious and life-threatening health problems, including liver damage that might be fatal. Cholesterol is important to life. The body would not make more of it unless it really needed to do so.

Depression, Chronic Fatigue Syndrome, Lupus, Multiple Sclerosis, Muscular Dystrophy

These conditions are caused by prolonged chronic dehydration. They will clear up once the body becomes well and regularly hydrated in conjunction with adequate intake of the essential intracellular mineral, mentioned above. In these conditions, exercising your muscles should be part of the treatment program. Among the letters that follow, you will come across reports of the healing power of water in the above conditions, whose mention would send shivers down your spine, let alone being saddled with their label.

For more information on the above topics you should read my other books, which are designed to give thorough explanation of the diseases caused by dehydration and how to reverse them. I recommend three of my books: *Your Body's Many Cries for Water; ABC of Asthma, Allergies, and Lupus; Water: For Health, For Healing, For Life.*

The rest of this book is dedicated to people's reports on how adjusting their daily water intake and sticking to the routine I have identified in my above books has reversed their serious health problems. In medical research, when studying chemical compounds and drugs, the custom has been to do double-blind studies to investigate the effectiveness of the compound. Such studies are *only* useful for comparative evaluation of foreign-to-the-body substances that might even kill the person when used in larger doses. In studying the effects of lifestyle changes and dietary manipulations, the methodology used is called "outcome studies" when the patient participates in the research by observing the markers of change and reporting the outcome. The stories you will read fall into this category of research.

When I discovered that water is a better natural medication for a host of disease conditions than anything the drug industry has to offer, I wrote the book *Your Body's Many Cries for Water* for the public. I asked my readers to report their personal observations on the way increased water intake improved or reversed their health problems. The letters that follow are some of the reports I have received. They are *not* "anecdotal reports." They are objective observations of people whose health problems had taken them to their doctors and were dragged through the sick-care system's maze of very expensive treatment rituals and procedures. These stories are all the more genuine and valid because no exchange of money was involved and no manufactured product stood to gain from the treatment process. They have been edited *only* to correct typographical errors; the words and, especially, the emotions belong to the writers. You have to be blind or a party to the drug industry's crime against society to brush aside these personal observations of individuals who noticed the reversal of the dis-ease process in themselves, or to dismiss their reports as merely "anecdotal."

Author's Recommendations

Warning: It is true that water is a medication in so many health problems of the human body, but too much water is just as dangerous as too much of any medication. Please do not try to reverse the serious problems of persistent and well-established dehydration of the body in one or two days. The human body is a complex chemical plant that *needs time,* and some additional primary ingredients, to achieve its prior normal state once again. The body is not like a car, the gas tank of which you can fill up without having to worry for the next few hundred miles. You need to understand the way the human body works. This is the reason you need to read more on the subject. This book is intended to show you the possibilities. To achieve these possibilities for yourself and become your own healer, you need to read my other books. They will show you how to tap into the new fountain of knowledge about water in order to simply and naturally achieve vibrant health and a longer, more productive and joyful life.

For God's sake, do not cut out your serious medications without sufficient caution and consultation with your physician, even if he is in the opposite camp. You need to coax him to read about and understand what dehydration is. Give him a copy of this book. We always need a second opinion to address our health problems. This is why you always need your doctor to be there for you. Once your doctor realizes where he/she has gone wrong, his/her sincerity to him/her oath as a physician will make him/her take your side.

My criticism of the "sick-care system" applies to the teaching establishments that perpetuate medical misinformation and the policymakers of the institutions within the system. Of course, it does not apply to the honorable and dedicated members of society who lovingly and selflessly serve the sick in medical establishments.

The Ultimate Truths in Medicine
The Healing Power of Water, a New Medical Knowledge

Duodenal Ulcer; Indigestion;
Colitis: Back Pain; Allergies;
Chronic Sinus Infection:

It has been one year since I first read your book, which was given to me as a present by Marcel Thevoz. Since then my health has improved significantly. I am now 52 and in excellent health. This was not the case before your book and Marcel's kindness inspired me to make water an integral part of my life.

To most people I was successful and in excellent health—normal weight, unusual strength and endurance, above average at sports, with an excellent diet (a lot of fresh vegetables and whole grains and very little meat, animal products or processed food). Yet my list of complaints stretches over the last fifty years and includes duodenal ulcer (age 19), indigestion, colon and elimination problems (age 19–51), food allergies (age 12–17), chronic sinus infections (age 5–51), chronic and acute back problems (age 13–51), emotional illness and mental confusion (age 6–51).

These problems were even more bewildering and confusing because I am intelligent, educated, and motivated to find solutions to problems. I have been searching for answers to these problems for 35 years. I have looked for answers in diet, diet supplementation, exercise, yoga, meditation, traditional religion, spiritual practices, acupuncture, traditional medicine, chiropractic, massage, Reike, polarity balancing, 12 step programs, and self-improvement books and courses such as EST and the Hoffman Quadrinity Process.

I had of course read many times about the importance of drinking plenty of water. I even invested in a reverse osmosis water filter six years ago hoping that the improved taste of the water would motivate me to drink more water. In spite of this, I never gave water therapy a fair chance. Until I read your book, other beverages always looked better to me, particularly tea and coffee.

At that time I read your book I had a chronic nerve injury in my upper back that intermittently prevented me from playing golf or racquetball for a period of two years. My arm strength was about 1/3 of what it had been only two years previously. I was at a low point in my life physically and mentally.

I have never been drunk in my life or smoked more than 5 cigarettes in a day. At that time I was not smoking or drinking any alcohol. Yet I found myself obsessed with thoughts of caffeine, smoking and drinking. Although I have been a frequent visitor at chiropractic, osteopathic and massage therapists, I had not needed to visit medical doctor in 15 years. In my desperation I went to an M.D. who prescribed an anti-stress medication, a pain reliever and a muscle relaxant. I took the prescribed doses and fell into a semicoma for 16 hours and discontinued the medication. A few weeks later Marcel came to my home for dinner and gave me your book.

Within one week of adding 2–3 quarts of water to my diet I noticed that:
- The pain from the nerve injury went away and I was able to begin exercising.
- I had much less indigestion and gas.
- My urges and compulsive behavior lessened substantially or vanished. I no longer had to fight the urge to smoke, drink, stuff myself or use excessive amounts of caffeine.
- My energy level improved.
- My thinking and work improved.

Please feel free to use me as a reference. I am happy to talk to anyone about water at any time.
Sincerely, W. E. G.

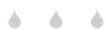

Back Pain:

I would like to thank you and share with you the significant progress I have enjoyed in the healing of my back. While reading your book, *Your*

Body's Many Cries for Water, I learned of your book, *How to Deal with Back Pain and Rheumatoid Joint Pain*. Following your suggested exercises—plus a few of my own—and drinking the amount of water you suggest as well, I am pleased to report that I have enjoyed much more strength and a lot less pain in my back.

I had a back injury well over twenty years ago, while helping to lift a piano for a friend. It seems that one of the disks in my lower back was crushed or badly damaged. It had gotten progressively worse over the years to a point a couple of years ago when it would go into spasms—rendering me unable to walk. The pain was excruciating. This would usually be triggered by a slight amount of lifting—especially front on. If I bent over and lifted something much over 10 pounds, I would be in trouble for some days.

Upon starting your suggested back exercise program about a year and a half ago, I saw slow but consistent progress. Last summer was the acid test. Ten and a half years ago, I retired as an atomic clock researcher in Boulder, CO, and bought a farm in central Utah—near my hometown and family. My wife and I have pretty much had others run the farm until this last summer, but circumstances arose that we needed to run it. This included moving 30-feet-long irrigation pipes, baling and hauling three crops of hay. The farm is not big enough to be modernized, so my sons and I with some hired help were hand lifting 90-pound bales of hay up on a truck and hay wagon—with hay leaves down my sweating neck and all. We had to also lift them into the hay barn—harvesting well over a thousand bales. Having been raised on a farm, I have never minded hard work and this was hard.

There is no way that I could have done that the year before, and it actually felt good to be able to do this hard work. I have always tried to keep myself in good physical condition, but some years ago I had to even stop jogging because it hurt my back too much. Now I can also run again without serious pain. Considering also that I am 66 years old, I feel that the whole thing is pretty remarkable and I thank you for the tremendous assist in my recovery. I am far from all the way better, but the trend is right and my back is getting stronger all the time. This morning and yesterday I shoveled about a foot of snow off of our walk with no significant back pain. I haven't been able to do that for years.

You suggested extra weights on the feet as one does the back exercises. I just wear shoes and have a three-pound weight in each hand to strengthen my upper body while I am at it. The extra exercises that I do in addition to yours are all toward strengthening the back muscles and for general cardiovascular and lymph system circulation improvement. These include: 1) lying on each side and doing scissors with my free arm and leg in circular motion as well as up and down; 2) sit ups and leg lifts while lying on my back; 3) push ups from the knees and the toes with particular emphasis on flexing and using the lower back muscles—activating the osmotic pumping of water action as you suggest for the lower back; 4) jumping jacks, touching the floor with the weights in my hands, and cross touching the right hand to the left foot while strad-dled, and vice-versa; 5) doing a variety of jumping exercises on a re-bounder, which is excellent for the lymph system circulation; and 6) then a variety of stretching exercises to keep the whole body limber. I add to these walking with my wife, cross-country skiing, and mountain bike riding every day when the weather permits. We can usually do one of these most days of the year.

It feels so good to feel good. Life has been really good to me, and a good health allows me to better serve and does those things that I feel are most important. I love to express my gratitude by serving, and you can't do that very well lying on your back in pain. Thanks again for helping so significantly to take that pain away. I was so impressed with your first book, that I did a book report and have it posted on my website: www.allanstime.com/Health/water.htm. Your second book is saving my back. My wife has found significant benefit from your water cure as well. Gratefully yours, D. W. A.

♦   ♦   ♦

Back Pain:

I was diagnosed with reflux (hiatus hernia) some years ago and treated with Prilosec medication. Recently I returned to the gastroenterologist since I was experiencing upper back pain at night. He ordered many tests and prescribed Prevacid. The tests all came back normal; but a year later, the pressure and pain in my upper back intensified. I returned to the doctor once again. He doubled up the medication (Prevacid) for two weeks and ordered more of the same tests. Once again, the tests came back negative. Yet, as the two weeks progressed, I felt worse. If two Prevacid pills a day didn't relieve the pain, I figured I might as well stop myself. It was at this time that I mentioned going off the medication to a doctor friend of mine. He said, "Helen, drink water." With that said, along came his dear wife with your book, *Your Body's Many Cries for Water*. I took it home with me to read. It was such a revelation and has changed my life. Although I never liked to drink water (and drank little of anything), I began incorporating it into my lifestyle. The pain in my back is gone!!

I shall forever be indebted to you. I hope to share this information with as many people as I can.
Sincerely, H. H.

Osteoporosis:

I was previously diagnosed with advanced osteoporosis and two collapsed vertebrae, which led to the loss of 3 inches in height. Since the diagnosis, I have done everything the doctors recommended to maintain the level of bone density I had and to prevent any further fractures, but I increased my water intake.

This week I had an appointment for a bone density test. During the test, the technician said the results didn't look right on the hip measurement and she decided to redo that portion of the test. (I think she could not believe her eyes because of the 17% increase.)

The doctor said that the test results revealed that there is a 10% increase in bone density in my back and a 17% increase in bone density in my hip. There has also been a gain of 1" in height.

This disease affects men and women. It is considered the 12th leading cause of death in the U.S. 1.3 million bone fractures are attributed to the condition annually.

Thank you so much for your book *Your Body's Many Cries for Water,* it certainly turned my life around.

Sincerely, C. M.

Note: Do not be surprised at the improvement in bone density as a result of adequate hydration of the body. The reason is very simple. Bone structure is also a repository of stored energy that the body can tap into when necessary. As you know, when you heat water, the dissolved calcium in the boiling water gets deposited as a film inside the kettle. It is the chemical property for one calcium atom to stick to another calcium atom when they are heated. Scientifically, each atom of calcium that sticks to another atom of calcium traps one unit of energy between them. The body has learned to separate the calcium bond and release the energy therein, equivalent of one ATP unit of energy for each bond.

Dehydration means low energy reserves in the body. As the body becomes more and more dehydrated, it is forced to break up its bone structure to tap into its stored energy. This is how people develop osteoporosis. Hydrating the body properly does the reverse. Water is the main source of energy to the human body. It produces "high heat of activation" at the cell membrane. It heats up the body and provides energy for all its chemical reactions. The body has learned to convert and store the energy of heat into chemical energy in the formation of ATP, and the excess of it is then stored in the calcium stores inside the cells and in the bones. This is the reason C. M. could reverse her tendency to develop osteoporosis. When you stimulate the "bone tissue" by putting weight on it, the bone-forming cells get stimulated to lay down bone and make the structure more dense, provided you have the available energy to fuse calcium atoms together. Water provides the extra energy for this action. Hence the 17 percent rise in CM's hip bone density.

◆   ◆   ◆

Constipation and Hemorrhoids;
Heartburn; Cold Feet and Hands;
Foul Urine Smell: Depression:

I was drinking two or more pots of coffee and a few sodas every day. No water. I am retired about three years now. While working I would drink some water from the cooler at work. Now that I am home I don't have a cooler and don't like tap water, so I drank none at all.

Symptoms:

- My urine was getting very strong. I thought I would need to see a doctor soon for a possible infection.
- My constipation was so bad I was using hemorrhoid preparation 2 to 3 times a week.
- My stomach burned sometimes so I used Tums a few times a month.
- Also I seemed to have some sort of bronchial problem, a deep cough, soreness and very thick phlegm.

During the winter it was necessary to wear long johns for the first time in my life. At night I needed socks, long johns and a T-shirt and I would cover up with a sheet and two blankets. I was so cold in the morning I would use a blow dryer to warm my feet, then after putting socks on I would warm the socks on my feet. Lastly, I would heat the shoes I was going to wear. It was common to be cold enough I could hardly function. It was painful. If I tried to go for a walk I would wear two pairs of gym pants.

I went to the gym and used the treadmill and cross trainer. I started feeling depressed when I got to the gym, didn't know why. My numbers had been slowly decreasing, that is the speed and inclination settings. I always hold the sides.

When I walked freely at the shopping mall my sides would hurt so badly it brought me to tears. My feet would hurt but the side pain overwhelmed this.

My karate lessons have been getting harder and harder. The number of moves, like kicks I could do, has been dropping regularly. The instructor wanted 25 to 50 kicks and we have been reducing this to 10 to 15, kept saying I was getting old, disregarding how fast I was aging in just a few years.

I had been trying to lose weight but if I cut back my food intake I would get cold and achy much like getting a cold. I was getting so uncomfortable I did not like to get up in the morning, just didn't feel good to sit or stand. I can understand how lack of enthusiasm or lethargy or even depression could set in.

One curious thing I noticed was on the skin of my hand. When I held my hand out the skin seemed like mummy skin, very dry. My hand was flat. I was starting to worry about my health, maybe diabetes. I have always tested fine for this and my web research did not seem to support anything I could find.

I know doctors tell you to drink water when ill so the strong urine caused me to start drinking water to flush my system. About the same time a friend sent me an email about dehydration. I was shocked to learn a few percent dehydration could cause a 10 to 20 percent drop in athletic output. This email led me to do research on the web. I was amazed to find I had almost all of the signs of dehydration. I decided to look for books and eventually found your book *Your Body's Many Cries for Water* at Amazon. I have been following the regime of 2 or more glasses first thing in the morning, one one-half hour before each meal, one 2 and a half hours after each meal and one at night. During the day I drink a little more, a glass or two. Also the coffee intake has been reduced.

Results:

- My urine no longer smells and the constipation has almost completely disappeared. I didn't know bowel movements were this easy, it's almost pleasant. My stomach is fine now and the bronchial discomfort is gone.

- I now sleep in just underwear just like years ago. I have had many nights when my legs felt so warm they almost felt sweaty. It's amazing how far off my body's temperature regulation had gotten. When I am exposed to cold it just feels cold, it doesn't hurt anymore.

- When I get up in the morning I feel fine. Sometimes I just enjoy sitting because I feel so good, no discomfort.

- When I drink 2 or 3 glasses when I first get up I get a lift from it similar to what we get from coffee. If I go on the computer in the morning the screen is brighter, seems to sparkle. I don't understand this but it happens.

- When I cut back on my eating to lose weight I just get hungry, not sick. I actually smile at this because I feel I have control. A little hunger but I can stand it.

- Regarding my hand. Now when I hold my hand out the blood vessels show and there are little muscle bumps all over. Before my hand was flat.

- I never feel depressed any more. I attribute this to just feeling better. Slight pain and/or discomfort slowly grind away at one's attitude.

Some problems slowly sneak up on a person and we don't notice the degradation or we adapt to it. The most directly measurable result is at the gym. Using the same speed and elevation settings as before, my heart rate is 10 to 12 points lower. At first I thought this was the machine but all the equipment shows this. Some of these fixes occurred very quickly, a few days; some took a month or two to completely take effect.

Overall, I am amazed at the influence of low water intake. I have clear-cut results and much optimism. My karate instructor now wants me to get my black belt. This seems amazing to do at 60 but I did have training in my 20s. He is sure I can do it and the system I am studying does not give the belts out easily like some do. This makes me feel very proud and has increased my self-esteem. It makes me want to do more things.

I read and reread your book often. Many of the things in your book I would not even believe a few months ago but I have proof. I highly recommend the book to everyone I know. I have become a water spokesman. There seem to be many examples among my friends especially the older ones. There are people over 50 that drink nothing but coffee, tea or alcohol and they have most of the symptoms I had. If I can just get them to cut back the coffee and drink water I am happy and feel I am helping. It is easy to imagine how dehydration can lead to serious disease. My informal data gathering seems to indicate a serious dehydration problem with the elderly, especially older men.

It is very clear your book is very valuable. My only criticism is I had to reread to find your daily routine for water consumption, wish you had this as a separate chapter or table. There is no question your book is a valuable service on an important topic, thank you very, very much. I also enjoyed your discussion on diet beverages though this was not one of my problems. As a matter of fact, the book is a must read, far more valuable for good health than possibly anything else on the shelf.

In one of the letters from readers of your book it was said he kept two books on his nightstand, the Bible and yours. At first I thought this was funny but you know what, your book may be that important. It has improved the quality of my life.
P. C. Van K.

**Vertigo; Cramps; Gum Separation;
Improved Autism:**

I was so pleased that you found my letter useful for your new edition, which I found very impressive. Thank you!

As you know I mentioned that by following your water routine I immediately noticed an improvement in my vertigo problem. Here is an update. Besides sleeping with one pillow instead of four, I can shampoo in a washbowl without getting dizzy. I can lie on a slant board, which elevates my feet 18 inches. I don't have to worry about turning my head quickly when driving. While vertigo was not a constant problem it had been with me from time to time for at least 40 years; but that is history now.

Some other benefits—I seldom have leg cramps now which bothered me almost nightly, and more good news, most of upper teeth are capped and over the years had developed unsightly gaps which were now gone and the gums looked as good as originally. What a happy surprise! That certainly emphasizes how the body tissues can dry out and shrink. For an 84-year-old, I am in very good health and in some ways better than 10 years ago.

Charles (who is deaf & autistic) is doing well. He has gained weight which he needed and looks healthier and behaves better than at any time since he was a toddler. I don't know whether I'm imagining it or not, but it seems to me he is responding to some sounds lately. I tell other people about drinking water whenever I can.

Thank you for your contribution to humanity and your courage and persistence in working for the acceptance of this information. I have seen references to your book in several health publications.
In appreciation, M. R.

**Migraine; Back Pain;
Increased Energy:**

My wife Carol and I will be forever grateful for showing us the most simple, economical way to better health. To think, all you have to do is to drink eight glasses of water and one quarter of a teaspoon of salt per quart per day. I now know that anyone who does this will notice considerable improvement in his or her health. I have yet to hear anyone who has taken that advice say they haven't noticed a difference. It works. You just have to do it. No one can do it for you. Also people who are looking for better health through water must be made aware of the variables. For every cup of coffee I drink, I also drink an added glass of water. For every glass of soda, I do the same. After a short time, you lose the taste for these other drinks. I remember the first time I drank diet soda I hated the taste. Because that's all my family used to buy, I started to acquire a taste for it, and then I hated the taste of regular soda. The same holds true when you start to drink water on a regular basis. Now I can't stand the taste of any soda.

I never would have thought the day would come when I would enjoy a tall glass of cold water with a pizza pie. That's right! I can't even drink soda with pizza. Water tastes much better. I still enjoy two cups of coffee in the morning, but I drink a glass of water before each cup. Some of the benefits we've reaped from taking your advice are 99% less back pain, a higher energy level, the absence of severe migraine headaches, and finally a thirst that needs quenching. For the past twenty years I never drank because I was thirsty; I drank because I believe drinking diet soda becomes habitual. Since I started drinking water, I found that I drink because I am actually thirsty and that alone amazes me.

I was diagnosed as having a herniated disc; I will never forget the pain that used to shoot down my legs if I moved the wrong way. There were times my wife had to put my socks on me in the morning. Then I would have to crawl out of bed. I couldn't sit in a chair, any kind of chair for six months. If I were standing when the pain hit, it would knock me right to the ground where I would stay until I could muster up the courage to crawl to the couch or bed. Sometimes I would just lie where I was for hours. To get to the doctor's I had to lie on my stomach in the car. I had to eat at the kitchen table standing up. Now don't get me wrong, the doctor helped me also, because the pills I took for inflammation helped at the time for a while; and I could not have endured without them.

Here's what I'm saying. The first year I had a prescription for the original bottle and three refills, all of which were used in one year. The second year I started drinking the water, and I used only one bottle of pills in one year. I really think I could have done without those pills the second year, but the pain was so horrendous it seemed as if I needed that little bit of extra insurance once in awhile if I felt the slightest twinge in my buttocks. (That's where the pain would always originate.) I'm convinced the pills eased the pain at the time, but the water aided in the cure.

The reason I say aided is because I also had to start walking and exercising. When I saw the big improvement in my health I almost naturally started eating more of the right foods. It seems as if everything starts falling into place once you make it a way of life. I'm not a health purist. I still smoke; but you know what? I smoke less now. I still don't live or breathe or eat every hour of the day in the way that's best, but, overall

I'm in much better health now than I was a couple of years ago. For the most part, everything in moderation never killed anyone. I even started bowling a couple of years ago. At one time I was convinced I would never be able to pick up a sixteen-pound bowling ball and throw it down an alley. I owe this new way of life to you Dr. Batmanghelidj. Thank you! I am writing you this letter in the hope other people will see it and maybe it will motivate them just enough to try it. If I help just one person, it will have been worth it, I am forever indebted to you.
H. J. F., Jr.

Chest Pain; Ulcers; Angina

I'm writing in response to your show on our radio station with Bob Butts. I have had a problem with ulcers, chest pain and angina for the past five or six years.

I am now drinking 2 quarts of water a day and have cut out caffeine, and it works!! We have been plugging your book on the air and hope to talk to you soon. Thank you for keeping me pain free.
Sincerely, J. D.

Back Pain; Neck Pain;
Carpal Tunnel; Energy Level:

Sometime before Christmas last year a friend in England called my home after 8 years of my not seeing him. My husband and I met Mike when we were touring England, Scotland and Ireland with a group of about a dozen people briefly in 1995 and Mike was the driver of our bus.

We talked a long time and during the conversation he told me of a couple of websites he thought I should visit after I told him the business we're in and that my husband had undergone by-pass surgery about a year ago. One of the sites he told about was www.watercure.com, which is yours. When I found the website, I ordered 5 copies of *Your Body's Many Cries for Water*, but immediately started drinking more water due to the bit I read on the site. The truth is, in the past I had drank more water than I was presently.

Now, let me tell you that I see a chiropractor regularly and have felt the need to for the last 25 years. I consider myself "healthy" as I have not had any major illness and I am not overweight, but I hurt all over and I did not look forward to aging because I thought as I got older I would only hurt more.

I broke my arm when I fell over a log at the beach walking backwards in May of 2001 and healed quickly and extremely well, but it seems that since the injury I have been having trouble with my wrists. The diagnosis of my chiropractor and the doctor who took care of my broken arm is carpal tunnel in my right wrist and de Quervain's disease in my left wrist. Seeking help has been quite expensive and after wearing the wrist braces and taking the ibuprofen in huge doses as prescribed by the medical doctor I had no relief. I did get some relief when my chiropractor adjusted my wrists, though it was only temporary.

When I got your book I immediately began to read it, searching for how much water to drink and when. I didn't find the answer early on as I read, but I finally put "the program" together as I neared the end of the book and jotted it down. My husband says I am on a "water kick" when I ask people if they drink a lot of water; but even he has begun to follow the "program" and he is doing better every day.

Today I am feeling so much better; I can say that I am looking forward to growing old "gracefully" I hope! I have more energy, my joints, back and neck feel so much better and my chiropractor says he feels the difference in my adjustments once a month. The aches are gone; my body does not hurt like before. Although I still have some discomfort in my wrists occasionally, the pain is gone. It's very easy to forget pain existed when it's gone but I can tell you I wept many times when my wrists hurt so bad it made me feel helpless. That pain is gone!!!

I will continue to tell everyone I can to drink more water and why; and let me add, in regards to my health, that I am only 57 years old. After many years of taking hormone therapy for menopausal symptoms and then stopping them, against my doctor's orders, I found that I am thinking more clearly; in retrospect I felt my head had been "foggy" for a long time. But since I have been doing the "water program" faithfully for about 4 months now I have been clear headed and have more energy as well. This thank you letter comes from my heart, your research is so beneficial and your solution is so simple and sensible.

I believe God created man and water. . . . He gave us the water because we need it!!
Sincerely, L. R.

$$\smwhitedot \quad \smwhitedot \quad \smwhitedot$$

Heart Attack; Chest Pain; Difficulty Sleeping; Memory Loss; Bladder Retention; Vision Problems:

It was in the spring of 1991 when I first learned from a member of the Foundation for the Simple in Medicine the value of water as a form of medication. Six months before, I had suffered two heart attacks and had undergone angioplasty surgery. After the operation, I was prescribed heavy dosages of calcium and beta-blockers, baby aspirin, nitroglycerine (for pain), and cholesterol-reducing medicine for recovery. The angiogram before the angioplasty had shown one of the arteries of my heart was 97 percent blocked by cholesterol deposits. I was told my heart had been damaged.

After six months of strict attention to my prescribed "recuperation" program, I noticed that my condition was rapidly deteriorating to the extent that I had difficulty sleeping because of pain in my left arm, back and chest, and also felt these same pains when I took my daily walks. I visualized myself going for bypass surgery at the scheduled time for reevaluation of my condition. By this time, I also suffered from serious side effects caused by the medications, such as: my prostrate created retention and blocking problems, I had also developed problems with my vision and memory recall.

I first began my rehabilitation through diet by a regular intake of six to eight 8-ounce glasses of water each day for three days. I was told to drink water a half-hour before eating my daily meals. I cut off my anti-cholesterol pills, aspirin and nitroglycerine pills. Judging by the effect of the water, it seemed I did not need them. I also started taking orange juice and started using salt in my diet again. (I had been on a sodium-free diet.) After the first three days, I was feeling more comfortable about all of that added water. After three weeks of gradually reducing the calcium and beta-blockers, I noticed some very favorable changes. Whenever I felt pain, I would drink water and get instant relief. My diet remained the same . . . . fruits, vegetables, chicken, fish, orange juice and carrot juice. To get more tryptophan, I was asked to add cottage cheese and lentil soup to my diet.

Dr. Batmanghelidj requested that I take two one-hour walks (25-minute mile) a day. After the second month, I noticed no more pain, even walking up steep hills. After the fifth month I changed my walks to 1/2 hour and increased my pace to a 15-minute mile. No constrictions were noticed during my walks and my energy had increased two-fold. Much of my power to recall had been re-established, and my vision returned to normal.

In October 1991, I had a series of chemical and physical tests, including x-rays, sonogram, echocardiogram and electro-cardiogram, to determine the state of my heart. The tests showed that my heart had restored to its normal state and I did not need any form of medication to cope with my daily routine. My doctor could not believe how simply all this change had taken place.
Thank you, J. O. F.

Note: J. O. F's recovery has been so dramatic that he asked me to publish this letter in my book with his name, address, and telephone number for people to contact him for guidance, should they wish to use the water cure program and avoid the knife-happy system. He was inundated with telephone calls. He coached many people to follow the program and achieve better health. People would call him at all hours without any consideration for his convenience. This continued until he had to change his telephone number. Eventually he must have moved from the address on his letter to achieve peace. He was well and symptom-free for the duration that you could contact him. J. O. F's experience is the reason the name, address, and telephone number of people whose letters are included in this book have been edited out, even when their authors wanted to be contacted.

WATER CURES DRUGS KILL

Angina:

I am 90 years old and I have angina. I do not get chest pains or cramps, but at the base of my throat I get an ache—a very painful tension and my pulse beats like a run-away horse.

But after reading your book *Your Body's Many Cries for Water*, I started drinking water. When I get an attack of angina, I rest and drink water. Would you believe it? I don't need the medication anymore. I am so glad, because the medication burned my mouth and gave me oral ulcers. Now I carry a small bottle of water with me at all times in addition to drinking it at home. Thanks a million!
Sincerely, L. J.

Massive Heart Attacks;
Extensive Heart Muscle Damage:

I am compelled to write to you to express my gratitude for who you are and how you have dramatically altered my life. The information contained in your seminal publication *Your Body's Many Cries for Water* has saved my life and allowed me to rebuild and repair heart muscle damage that was pronounced irreparable. With proper hydration, I have fully recuperated and once again lead a full and active life. Please share my story with others so they too might know that full recovery is not just a dream, it is a real possibility!

My name is Oleg Yasko. I am a doctor of naturopathy and a certified nutritional consultant. I am 49 years of age and currently reside with my family in Brooklyn, NY. I own and operate a clinic dedicated to the practice of Holistic Integrative Health.

I was born and raised in Kiev, Union of Soviet Socialist Republics, and received a master's degree in biochemistry from University of Kiev, 1972. My family immigrated to the United States in 1979.
In 1985, at the young age of 33, I suffered a massive heart attack in Albany, NY. At that instant I knew there would be no denying my line-

age. My father had suffered a series of heart attacks, with the third one fatal at the age of 61. My brother had a heart attack at age 36, and at age 43 the second occurrence also proved fatal. I was now brought face to face with my fate.

I consulted with all the traditional medical sources, and they could only point to the immediate causation, occluded arteries. They offered neither remedy nor adequate explanation of the genesis of this occlusion. I was a young man who had been a champion wrestler and was in the active military for many years. I considered myself in excellent physical condition. I discounted the explanation of genetic causation, and began my own search for answers.

This search seemed to arrive at a dead end when in March of 1997 I suffered yet another massive coronary. At this juncture I was informed that over 44% of my heart muscle was compromised, and the prognosis for any sort of complete recovery was termed negligible.

As I convalesced, more uncertain than ever about ever finding a resolution to my dilemma, a friend passed me a copy of a book *Your Body's Many Cries for Water*. This book would save my life!!!

This book stated the hypothesis that prolonged severe dehydration had caused the major coronary arteries to become brittle. The resultant cholesterol buildup in the arterial lining was the body's natural attempt to protect the artery from further damage. Unfortunately this buildup also restricted the blood flow sufficiently to cause myocardial infarction—twice.

Immediate testing determined that I was indeed severely dehydrated. My search now took a more focused path, to resolve my state of constant dehydration that had contributed to these attacks and to somehow rebuild my damaged heart muscles.

It was these efforts to resolve this chronic dehydrated condition that led me to understand the vital role that proper hydration played in our bio-system. A role that slowly but certainly allowed my heart muscles to recuperate fully even after two major heart attacks and the considered prognosis from the physicians I consulted with that my heart was irreparably damaged.

I am pleased to report that I am alive, healthy, hydrated and practicing my profession as a healer with renewed enthusiasm and vigor.

Thank you Dr. Batmanghelidj for your courage and persistence in disseminating your message worldwide that dehydration is indeed the primary foundational cause, as well as rehydration a foundational remedy, for many health problems of the human body.
Sincerely, Dr. Oleg Yasko

Note: I met Dr. Yasko at a conference in Arizona. I did not know he had suffered two massive heart attacks until he told me his story. When I met him, he was active, vibrant, and full of joyful enthusiasm for his newly discovered natural remedy for many of our prevalent health problems. Indeed, he was so enthusiastic that he had initiated the conference—hence my invitation to speak.

The way I see it, the future of medicine in advanced societies will become transformed when healers like Dr. Yasko take over from the allopathic doctors who are mostly brainwashed by their system of university education and seem to be mentally programmed to serve the drug industry without hesitation. They just blurt out "double blind" and continue to dispense drugs that are known to be very toxic, to the point of making millions of people sicker—and even killing more than a hundred thousand trusting people every year.

◆   ◆   ◆

Asthma:

I will write you a formal letter but I wanted to thank you for your water cure. I have suffered with asthma for the last five years and have tried many natural ways to get rid of it or at least to get improvement. I have needed the inhaler at least two times per day and would wake up wheezing pretty near every morning. I did your cure for two weeks but still drank green tea (I love my caffeine); it did not work. I quit tea last Sunday and the asthma cleared up immediately. I only need the inhaler for hard exercise (ju jitsu class), and I wake up with no wheezing and no need for medication. I even put the water cure on our web site, as I am so impressed even at this early time. I know you are onto something.

Thank you, and I am telling all of my family.
Thank you, N. B.

◆   ◆   ◆

Obesity; Diet Sodas:

My mother asked that I write to you and tell you about my recent weight loss success. I know that I could have a much more successful loss if I would follow your formula and curb my eating habits, along with starting a regular routine of exercise. However just getting myself to get off 6 to 8 cans of Mountain Dew a day is a miracle in itself.

Within the last 9 months to a year, I have successfully been able to keep 35 excess pounds of baggage off. I am able to wear clothes that I thought would never touch my body again. I also have just about reached my goal size for my upcoming wedding. Even my fiancé had to admit that I am looking much better than when he first met me five years ago.

My success has been contributed to faithfully drinking half my body weight in ounces in water every day. Wherever I go, so does my water. To work, shopping, even my long 7-hour long car rides. That does make for a lot of rest area stops, but they are worth it. I do treat myself to an occasional mineral water or beer when I go out, but I have usually gotten my quota of water in for the day.

One interesting thing that I have noticed however is that once I have finished drinking my quota of water, I have absolutely no desire to drink anymore. Also I have found that I'm not thirsty anymore and it will usually take me awhile to drink some other type of beverage, whether it is juice, milk, beer, mineral water, etc.

I am looking forward to October 1st which is my wedding day, when I can walk down the aisle looking better than I have looked in 15 years, since I graduated from high school. It will also be nice to put my weight on my new driver's license without having to cringe for the first time. Thanks for the smaller me, D. M. G!!!!!

Note: D. M. G. has been married for a number of years. She has kids, and last I heard she seemed not to have weight problems anymore.

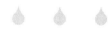

Asthma:

We passed on the information that you gave on your tape about asthma to a friend who had been to Mexico for a cure and had tried all the drugs for asthma. He usually ends up in the hospital about once a month, but the last couple of times he tried the water and salt, his symptoms were relieved rather quickly. Thank you for sharing your knowledge on water.
Gratefully yours, M. P.

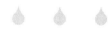

Asthma:

Thank you so much for your book. I've had asthma for nearly forty years and finally experienced marked relief with increased salt and water intake.
Thanks again, C. E.

Irritable Bowel; Stomach Pains;
Heartburn:

Shortly after my husband and I moved to the desert in Tucson, Arizona, in 1987, he began to complain of stomach pains. Of course we went to the doctor and he came up with the answer, irritable bowel syndrome. I'm sure they gave him something to take, but it is about 12 years ago and don't remember what it was but it did not help. He continued to complain to the doctor and after tests looking into his abdominal area and up his colon, finding nothing wrong, he was told it was all in his head. To make a long story short, by the beginning of 1999, the pain reached the point that he could not eat and was losing weight, went down to 112 lbs. The doctors, including specialists, came up with the same answer and they gave him anti-stress medicine. Finally the pain got so bad my husband asked me to take him to the hospital. Knowing they would probably want to do an exploratory which many people never come out of, I phoned a nutritionist friend of ours and he told me to give my husband two glasses of water, within 20 minutes and if the pain persisted give him another glass. Hurray it worked! I did not have to give him the third glass of water. My husband, a terrible skeptic, became a believer. He knows if the slightest pain comes back he didn't drink enough water that day. Not only did it take the pain away, but also his heartburn. I am telling family, friends and anyone I meet about the water cure and it has helped many of those whom I told.
Thanks for listening. Mrs. M. G.

Angina; Hiatal Hernia:

Just a short letter to thank you for informing our listeners about the health benefits of drinking two quarts of water a day.

Not only did you help our radio audience, but also I personally have enjoyed a resurgence of energy after drinking two quarts of water each day for just over one week.

The angina pain I endured for five years has disappeared and my distress from hiatal hernia has greatly lessened. I feel like a new person. I've been doing talk shows at xxx radio for the past 20 years, and I must say your interview with us is one I'll always remember.
Sincerely, xxx Broadcasting Corporation
S. M. L., Program Director

Note: This letter was written in 1994. Nine years later, in 2003, S. M. L. is well and totally cured of his initial problems.

◆　◆　◆

Migraine; Whiplash; Allergies; Weight Loss

Thank you for your book *Your Body's Many Cries for Water*. I have purchased copies for my children as they are all dehydrated and need water. But they look at me as if I'm crazy—even after seeing their mother and how she has lost weight, cured a whiplash neck problem she has had for over 20 years, cured a migraine headache problem she has suffered from for 20 years also. My wife also no longer suffers from allergies, and I could go on and on. We are both eternally grateful to you for this knowledge.

It's too bad people think it can't work because it's too simple and free. I have been diagnosed with benign prostate gland and have difficulty getting to sleep at night, so the temptation to cut back on my water intake is always there. Is there something I can do to solve my problem?
Sincerely, D. P.

◆　◆　◆

Back Pain; Hip Joint Pain:

I enjoyed our talk this morning. Thank you for taking the time to answer my questions. As I mentioned to you, about a year ago I began drinking 2–3 quarts of water daily. My intake up to this point had been 2 or 3 glasses daily, at most, offset by 4 or 5 cups of tea.

In February of 1996, my major problems were recurring lower back pain and severe hip joint pain; also my fingers had become painful in the joints. I had seen countless physicians over the years in dealing with my back. Even with proper nutrition & stretching exercises performed daily, the back would go out several times a year. Each time I would be in pain for several weeks before returning to normal.

After several months of drinking eight 8 oz glasses of water a day I felt really fit. One day a truck delivered some Belgian block stones—about 3 tons. The blocks each weighing about 10 lbs had been dumped on the lawn. My plan had been to get someone to lay them out as a border to the driveway, but for some reason I chose to try it myself. Normally I would watch carefully how I lift—bending the knees & squatting with straight back. This time I recklessly abandoned this conservative technique and bent over lifting each stone, as I would have 30 years ago. Something inside me encouraged me to do this—it was almost a test trial. I got the job done in 2 hours. There was little stiffness the next day and the dreaded back problem never materialized. Somehow, I knew it wouldn't.

This is the first year in 20 years I have no lower back pain. I am 64 and this is a joy. Also my hip & finger joint pains have vanished. My sense of smell is acute, better than I can remember ever.

I take this opportunity to tell people this water secret but sadly I do not succeed in convincing them. Most of the reactions are skeptical as if to say how could something free produce these results. I know for the most part the people I tell will be curious and experiment a bit but will never fully & seriously undertake the true change of habits necessary for success.

You are performing a good and valuable service in your crusade for sanity in medicine particularly as it applies to water. How true it is that often the most dramatic cures are the simplest if we will but have the faith to carry them out with perseverance.

Good luck and may God bless your efforts.
Best wishes, L. R.
New Zealand

Back Pain:

Thank you for writing the book *Your Body's Many Cries for Water.* I am a 75-year-old lady who has suffered with back pain for almost half my life, in spite of painkillers from my G.P., acupuncture, osteopathic treatment, chiropractic treatment, and a dozen other alternative treatments. I also suffered with swollen ankles and some other minor ailments. Now, after just a week on the water cure, I feel a tremendous difference in general health, and the back pain has greatly diminished—not gone, but sufficiently improved, to move me to write to you and tell you.

It was arranged some time ago that I should have an ultrasonic scan, which I will still have, but now much more hopefully. I will write again after the scan in a month's time to let you know how I'm faring.

Again, thank you for writing the book.
Very sincerely yours, R. G.

Back Pain:

I have had back problems ever since I sustained a sports injury in high school. During the ensuing years, I have had to have chiropractic treatment every so often to be able to work.

The last ten years I have had to have chiropractic treatment on a monthly basis and last summer my sciatic nerve gave me so much pain that I required weekly treatment and even that only partially solved the problem. After reading your book, *Your Body's Many Cries for Water,* I started drinking 8–10 glasses of excellent quality spring water together with at least 1/2 teaspoon of salt a day and since December 1, 1993, I have been able to walk without a limp or pain and have not had to visit a chiropractor in the last eight months.

It would be foolish for me to say that my 75-year-old degenerated back is good as new but the improvement and pain free ability to walk normally again is truly remarkable.
Sincerely, Mr. B. H. A.

◊   ◊   ◊

Shoulder, Back, and Neck Pain:
Weight Loss:

This letter is in reference to the book that I ordered from you in July 1996, Your *Body's Many Cries for Water.* I am astonished and greatly amazed at the effects that I have encountered from increasing my water intake on a daily basis.

I thought I was drinking enough water at one (1) quart daily, but after reading your book, I have increased my water intake from one to 3 quarts every day (sometimes more with my workouts). The benefits that I have received are beyond words; and they are:

Shoulder, back and neck pain that my doctors said that I would suffer with for the rest of my life are completely gone. I have lost weight. My skin has a rich glow and is extremely toned.

I could go on and on, but I just wanted to let you know that I am very glad that I found out about your book, was able to order it and not only for me, but have passed your information on to many others, and they are now drinking more water.

Thank you so much for your valuable information and keep up the good work.
Sincerely, R. B. F.

Numbness and Loss of Skin Feeling:

During the afternoon a few weeks ago, I was resting a few moments and felt a funny sensation in the forearm of my right arm. It was not a pain but numbing sensation. The numbing spread throughout my entire arm and lasted about fifteen minutes. When the numbing went away, I wondered what it was but figured it wouldn't happen again. Well, around 8 P.M. that night the numbing came back and lasted until 10 P.M. at which time I fell asleep. I was quite concerned and a little frightened. I didn't know what it was. When I awoke the next morning, my right arm still felt numb.

At this point, I was near panic. I called my parents and they agreed that if I called the doctor, he would put me in the hospital immediately. All I could think of was the expense of medical care and missing work and wondering what was wrong with me. My father said to wait until Monday (it was Friday A.M.) and if it was still there, to go to the doctor. My mother told me to go immediately. I thought perhaps it was a blood clot or clogged artery, and was really upset at the prospects of what faced me.

Then I called Fereydoon to see if perhaps I needed to drink more water or something, because he has a theory that water can cure many ailments. Instead of prescribing water, he asked questions about my anxiety level, diet, exercise, etc. I appreciate the fact that he takes this holistic approach to medicine, which is something most doctors do not do. After listening to my answers, he told me not to worry and prescribed a neck exercise I was to do six times during the day. I believe he said it was a pinched nerve or something. Anyway, I faithfully completed the exercises as prescribed. Friday evening the numbing seemed to be going away, and by Saturday morning I was completely healed. Fereydoon called me Saturday to see how I was doing, which I thought was really nice. He was very comforting and seemed to care, which meant a lot to me. He also called me a few times again later to make sure I was OK.

I thank the Lord Jesus for giving Fereydoon the wisdom and insight to solve my problem, because He is indeed the Lord that heals us.

I was one happy person, to have received the healing. To have your health is a blessing and something we should never take for granted. Thank you again Fereydoon. V. L.

Back Pain:

Thanks be to God for the restoration of ancient truth of the healing touch of water, which you, His servant, have brought to us.

I am a retired clergyman, having served the church for over forty years. Mostly small, rural churches have been my several callings. Not having large salaries, I have had to search for other activities to sustain me in later years. These were mostly physical. So it happened that my back had been injured.

Recently, back pain was the worst. I couldn't get out of bed without an attack. My wife had to put on my socks and shoes. Each step had to be taken slowly and carefully. Getting into the car was a problem. Pillow as a backrest was not very helpful.

In our retirement, my wife and I exhibit at craft shows; some of these are hundreds of miles to the neighboring state. We need to be on our feet eleven-plus hours each day from two to seven days.

Since I read your book in the first part of October, I began the regimen. Now it has been several weeks since I have been without pain. I have driven long distances; I have been on my feet twelve hours for several days, have carried big boxes, and have mowed our 15,000 sq. ft. lawn and I have done other strenuous yard work. My back is better than it has been for years.

Feeling that every one needs to know about this Godsend of water and salt, I am spreading the word every time I can to sufferers. My wife, Doris, and I meet relatives at craft shows who have the symptoms of dehydration. We've written letters to the editors of several local papers, requested our local bookstore to stock your book and bought extra books to personally distribute.

Yours truly, The Rev. F. E. O.

Neck Pain; Back Pain;
Joint Pain:

Recently I was encouraged by my chiropractor to read your book and listen to your tapes. I have been on the water treatment program for four months and I would like to share my progress.

For the first 48 years of my life I only drank a glass or two of water a week. I had heard all my life that one should drink eight glasses of water a day but I never took this information seriously. To me, 8 glasses of water seemed to be a ridiculously large amount. About three years ago I began a supplement program and began drinking more water. I tried to drink eight glasses a day, which I thought was a huge improvement. I felt that 4–6 glasses a day was helping my body and that I didn't need to push myself to 8–10 glasses a day. During my 4–6 glasses a day stint I was relieved of constipation and hemorrhoids.

Because of a car accident, I suffer from neck and back pain. It is not severe and I have an excellent chiropractor that keeps me relatively pain free. However, I had stiffness in my neck most days and recently had developed back and joint pain. Again nothing severe but I was beginning to worry about how much pain I would be in when I was in my 60s and upward. I eat well and faithfully take my supplements. Luckily, my chiropractor, Dr. Christine Jones, kept reminding me about the importance of water. She even lent me your book but I still didn't "get it." She finally lent me your tapes and I can say now that I "got it" in a big way!!

I started faithfully drinking 8 glasses of water a day. After a few days my joint pain started to disappear in both my elbows and my left knee. Around the fourth or fifth day I began to have what I call a sinus attack. I have had these all my life. I start to sneeze, become unable to breathe through my nose, my sinuses swell, there is terrible itching throughout my nose and sinuses and I am generally miserable and bedridden for four to five days. Sometimes this affliction will develop into a sinus infection and I then must take antibiotics. I try to avoid this because I believe antibiotics are very bad for the body.

I kept thinking about what I had heard you say on your tapes and started drinking more water even though I had already reached my two quarts for the day. I drank a glass of water every time my nose started to tingle as if I was about to start sneezing. The water seemed to keep me from having a sneezing fit. When I have these attacks, I can't sleep. I am unable to breathe properly and am generally restless and miserable. Because of this I was lying on the couch hoping that the TV would distract me. Around 1:00 A.M. I woke up surprised that I had fallen asleep. I realized that I had drifted off to sleep around 11:00 P.M. because I was breathing much, much better. I went to bed and awoke the next morning perfectly fine! You have no idea how thrilling this experience was for me.

After four weeks my joint pain in my elbows and knee was 80% gone, my lower back that had been bothering me for about six months was also about 80% better. My fingernails are free of fungus infection that I had been battling for years.

Thank you so much for your valuable information. It has changed my life in so many ways. I now have very little neck pain, no joint pain, no hemorrhoids, no lower back pain, my skin looks better, my eyes are not suffering from dryness, I have not experienced one allergy attack all spring and summer, my indigestion is gone and my fingernails look great. Blessings to you, K. K.

Knee Injury;
Medial Meniscus Tear:

I thoroughly enjoyed your Wilkes-Barre seminar and commented to my friend that it was the most interesting evening I had experienced in a long time. During the question and answer period, I explained to you my experience with a knee injury, but with this letter I hope to bring more detail and my reasoning in the matter.

On October 7, 1993, while running playing tennis, I injured my left knee; I heard a pop and squish and could no longer bend the knee.

Fortunately I did not fall to the ground. I was able to hang onto the net between the courts. Because of the pain, I painfully hobbled to my car and drove to my chiropractor thinking he might be able to help. He worked on the knee for more than an hour with ultrasound and I still felt no improvement. Once again, it was excruciating to get in and out of my car, but I did manage and finally arrived home at about 8:30 that evening. I hobbled up to bed and took Excedrin for the pain and tried sleeping without much success.

The next morning it was even more painful so my husband drove me to the knee center in Wilkes-Barre for an examination and what we thought would be arthroscopic surgery. Dr. Cooper referred me to the MRI Center for diagnosis and they reported that I had a bucket handle tear of the lateral meniscus. Dr. Cooper suggested that surgery should be a last resort because of the diversity of complications possible. He suggested that I stay off my feet as much as possible, but could go to work and do light things around the house.

As long as I kept the left knee straight, I didn't experience intense pain, but I limped for months. I went up and down stairs one step at a time for months. I returned to limited tennis playing about three months later but was unable to run. After playing tennis, I had to wrap my knee in an ice wrap for half an hour because of the pain. The doctor prescribed two weeks of physical therapy that helped some. After about four months, I began to get the courage to try running during tennis. I could do most activities, but frequently when I ran I would get a sharp pain at the side of my knee. Thank God the body knows instinctively how to help itself and if I would raise my left foot up to my knee four or five times the pain would go away. At that point, I felt fortunate that I had found something to ease what I felt would be chronic knee pain.

My therapy continued for all of 1994 and in January of 1995, I read an article in the *Metro* about the therapeutic effects of water. I purchased *Your Body's Many Cries for Water* and it made sense to me. On page 45 you show a well-hydrated and a dehydrated joint comparison, and even though I was drinking close to two quarts of water a day, I reasoned that my knee pain was probably caused because the knee cartilage was not sufficiently hydrated because it was thinner and somewhat brittle, it had a tendency to get caught between the bones during certain knee motions. It was at that time that I decided to increase my water intake to three quarts a day. After several weeks of the increased water intake, I was able to run again. I can even do squats without any pain, and it is wonderful to play a vigorous game of tennis with no fear of pain, thanks only to your Water Cure.

I very much believe that water, proper nutrition, exercise, fresh air, a positive altruistic attitude and the nutrient of natural daylight and sunlight are the most effective therapies for good health and best of all, they are free; and the only side effects are a sense of accomplishment and well being.

Thanks for your help and hope this letter will be helpful to others. Sincerely, E. D.

♦   ♦   ♦

Urinary Incontinence:

July 25, 1999 I had to go home from work because the pain in my knee became unbearable. (This was an old wound years ago caused by a chiropractor that had been bruised again.) I was staying in bed a lot, as it was too painful to walk.

Thank God Global Health Solutions got my name and address from somewhere, and I got your books and tapes (*Your Body's Many Cries for Water*). By July 3, 1999, I decided to try and walk around the block. I made it and July 4, 1999, I walked six blocks to church. On July 5, 1999, I rode seven hours only stopping twice to use the restroom (I have a very weak bladder and had even taken spare clothing as I was sure they would be needed). I arrived with not a drop of anything on my clothing and for the first time in my life I was not tired and I even took a walk before I went to bed.

I was very thin and was very limited in what I could eat. Suddenly I find myself eating things I have not been able to eat in years (peaches, cantaloupe, watermelon, tomatoes, cucumbers, pineapple and even sweets), and was enjoying them with no side effects.

I had not been drinking anything but water for years, but I had taken myself off salt. A bad mistake! My muscles were really screaming as well as many parts of my body.

I still have problems to be worked out, but I'm learning how to listen to my body and I hope to see the day I won't have any more problems with gas, digestion, swelling and circulation or allergies. I can truthfully say most days I do feel better than I have in many years and I can never thank you enough for your help.

May God bless you as you try to help those He has placed on this Earth. Gratefully yours, D. R.

Rheumatoid Joint Pain:

I have been suffering with rheumatoid arthritis pain. The pain in my joints was so severe I could hardly walk. I had spent so much time, energy and now most of the money I had saved, and still I was in pain. I had read about *Your Body's Many Cries for Water* some time ago, and I remembered it was very good, but until recently when a friend suggested that I read your book on rheumatoid arthritis and back pain, did I remember how potent the water cure could be. I started having most of the joint problems after I moved to the high desert. I didn't drink much water before I moved, and in the last two years, I have not increased my intake of water. After I read the book, I started drinking water in the A.M., two glasses a half hour before a meal, and then more water two hours after. I find I have usually had problems drinking water, but now, the more I drink, the more I want, and I am recognizing my so-called hunger as thirst. For the first time in 2 years, I am once again able to walk over a mile at a time. I am experiencing less and less pain and swelling in my ankles, knees, wrists, and other joints. I am 30 lbs overweight, and hope that being able to walk and move will help this situation as well.
Thank you, R. C.

Ankylosing Spondylitis:

Heroes are hard to find today, but I've found mine. As a victim of arthritis, and how I got rid of mine, please consider the natural remedy that healed me. Perhaps you too will find your hero.

I am a 58-year-old Anglo-Saxon male, who has suffered from rheumatoid arthritis of the spine. The medical people call it ankylosing spondylitis. It is a painful inflammatory malady, which eventually causes the spine to fuse in a stooped position. This severely debilitating arthritis has plagued me since my teenage years and was diagnosed as my main problem by the Mayo Clinic in Rochester, MN, back in 1967 when I was 30 years old. They told me there was no cure for ankylosing spondylitis. They recommended back exercises to strengthen my back muscles, and a light-bulb-powered heat tent to help alleviate the pain associated with the flare-ups. An attack can last for several weeks, and can locate anywhere on the spinal column. Extended stooping, heavy lifting, cold drafts and weather changes always aggravated my fragile condition. Because of my out-of-doors vocation in the wholesale minnow business, I could not avoid the things that aggravated my arthritic condition.

Eventually, after 20 years of suffering with the continuing pain, I could not take it any more. I sold my business and retired in 1976. My condition improved somewhat because I avoided the heavy workload. Severe spinal flare-ups occurred about once a month or whenever I did heavy lifting or stooped over during gardening. My sister-in-law used to call me the "walking comma" during gardening season: that's how crooked I became, especially during strawberry season. After an hour of picking strawberries, I used to have to lie on the ground on my back for several minutes just to straighten my back enough so I could get back to my car without crawling! During my suffering years the doctors had tried cortisone and aspirin to help me with my pain, but to no avail. Even massive doses of various vitamins and minerals recommended by friends did nothing for me. Always in the back of my mind was the Mayo Clinic diagnosis: there is no cure!

In February 1995, my painful journey was about to end. Another friend gave me a booklet from the University of Natural Healing, which featured an interview with a Dr. Fereydoon Batmanghelidj. He is a medical doctor originally from Iran. The doctor expounded on the fact that a great many chronic diseases are nothing more than symptoms of dehydration, or simply put, people not drinking enough water. I found Dr. Batman's claims astonishing but intriguing. When I read his explanation of the hydraulics of the spinal column and how dehydration compresses the discs, causing back pain, I decided to try his remedy because, frankly, I'm very wary of high-priced "cures," and drinking lots of water was an inexpensive way to experiment with his remedy.

Believe me, it was not easy to drink the required water each day, simply because I had not been a big water drinker. In fact, it was a rare occasion when I would drink even one glass of pure water. I always preferred coffee, tea or colas. Within one month of starting the water-drinking procedure, I was absolutely symptom free and beginning to think Dr. Batman was right! As I write this, 14 months have passed since I started the water regimen. I've had no relapse and remain pain free and have started to enjoy life again. It is now great to be alive and who knows, I may go back to work.

Thank God for Dr. Batmanghelidj's information and his book *Your Body's Many Cries for Water*. I recommend it highly. Dr. Batman's prescription for good health follows for those willing to try something natural and simple. If you suffer from ulcers, asthma, high blood pressure, high cholesterol, back and joint pain (arthritis), chronic fatigue syndrome, breast cancer, impotency, overweight problems, stress or depression, please try the water regimen for a few months and experience what being hydrated can do for your health. Dr. Batman also reminds us to make sure that you have at least 1/2 teaspoon of salt per day in your food intake to help your body utilize the added water consumption. The salt is crucial to the program.

I consider Dr. Batman's information as God-sent. He is my hero. It is my prayer that you too will benefit from his pain-relieving revelations on water.
Sincerely, L. P.

Hand Aches and Pains:

I first read about you in *Acres USA* journal and have told hundreds of my clients (I'm a massage therapist) to buy your book. Many have as the Doubleday Bookstore had to order LOTs of the *Many Cries* book to keep up with the demand. Whenever my hands ache I review my previous day's water intake and realize I was lacking in the 64 ounces. So I immediately drink 16 to 24 ounces at one sitting and 30 minutes later the aches in my joints and hands disappears. Further proof that you are 100% correct. If I ever have opportunity to speak personally to the President of the U.S. I will tell him he needs to publicly recognize you for your research. Keep at it, one day we will prevail over those who are so ignorant about the role of water in the body. Question, do you ever do any speaking engagements publicly? Or, do you prefer to do your work via writing, website etc. Thanks, J.

💧   💧   💧

Note: Unlike all the other letters which have been edited *only* for their names to protect people from excessive calls, I use Drew's full name in the letter that follows to leave no doubt that such a person does exist. He lives in New York and is now studying Chinese medicine. Drew Bauman's history of illness is unique in the way it illustrates the sequence of physiological events that take place when the body becomes persistently dehydrated. When you read the letter, you will begin to realize the connection between so many "disease conditions" and gradually establishing dehydration, and, more importantly, the emerging connection of major health issues to one another.

In him, the dehydration of early childhood revealed itself in the form of allergies and proceeded to manifest as diabetes, asthma, immune suppression and repeated infections, vascular disease, and eventually cutaneous B-cell lymphoma. In the established trends of modern medicine, Drew had to go from one doctor to another and one hospital to another for the symptomatic treatment of his various health problems. Ultimately, his treatment included being X-ray-roasted and he sustained extensive burns. Until he refused further treatment, they wanted to continue his X-ray-roasting to kill his cancer cells. Fortunately he realized that he would more readily die from his treatment protocol than from his variety of health problems.

About two weeks ago (April 2003), I received an elated call from Drew. He has just undergone extensive examination and investigation to see if he is still cancer-free. He got a clean bill of health. His "traditional" doctors were flummoxed and wanted to know how he had done it. Apparently, it is unheard of for his kind of lymphoma not to recur in six years. He proceeded to explain to them the water cure protocol! Here is the detailed history of his dehydration diseases.

Let me also explain the reason why Drew was contracting so many infections. Histamine is the primary water regulator of the body. It is also a primary immune system regulator. But when histamine gets engaged in water regulation of the body, it automatically suppresses the immune system at the bone marrow level of activity. It has to do it; otherwise dehydration would constantly cause immune system flare-up. This is the natural design of the body to conserve the immune system for serious infections and not waste its resources when the body is dehydrated.

Lymphoma; Allergies; Asthma;
Diabetes; Immune System Suppression
Diabetic Neuropathy:

My name is Andrew J. Bauman, IV, and I am 42 years young, yet at age 34 I felt and looked like I was at least 44! Most of my life has been spent battling illness and disease, whereas now I celebrate each moment of each day with a renewed vigor and vitality. I used to be chronically dehydrated and now I know better.

I was born on October 29, 1956, in Taylor, PA, in a small hospital near Scranton in Northeast Pennsylvania. My parents lovingly cared for me—including having me vaccinated. I was reared on infant formula and later cereal, juices, and a small amount of water when I would cry from colic. After my first polio vaccine, I became mysteriously paralyzed from the waist down. Specialists were puzzled, yet diagnosed "Aborted Polio." It left as suddenly as it appeared. When I received a booster dose of the vaccine at around age 5 in first grade, the paralysis returned. Months of hospitalization and bed rest resulted in my gaining weight. I mostly ate my meals and had visitors, drank soda and some water now and then—and once again the paralysis disappeared.

When I began third grade—around eight years old—my allergic afflictions and symptoms had begun. I had problems with frequent dry coughs. I began experiencing some difficulties with breathing, itchy and watery eyes, and fatigue when I was around fresh-cut lawns from springtime until autumn. When I was a junior in high school, I experienced blackouts from allergies. Sometime around 1979, I saw a specialist who did testing and diagnosed me with allergies and asthma. I was approximately 23 years old. I was treated with allergy shots and inhalers. The treatments just seemed to make things worse. My lips were always dry and cracked. At that time of my life I was drinking about 2 to 4 cups of coffee per day along with a few glasses of soda and some tea and alcohol. I would have an occasional glass of water during the day. The allergies and asthma stayed with me until 1996 when my water intake was up to about two to three quarts a day. I no longer struggle with allergies or asthma.

My problems with diabetes began at age 14. I was diagnosed as an insulin-dependent or "juvenile diabetic." It was then that I began drinking diet beverages including those with caffeine. My water intake at that time was still only around 2 to 4 glasses a day and I was drinking tea and started drinking coffee. The diabetes resulted in many hospitalizations over the years. By the mid 1980s I had problems with diabetic neuropathy that was causing my legs to swell. I was scheduled to have dye injected into my legs to perform a diagnostic scan after a Doppler radar study showed some apparent blockages in the veins on my legs. The dye injections caused my veins to burst, which made the swelling worse. I was then diagnosed with "venous insufficiency." In 1994, I was told that my legs would probably have to be amputated within a year or so.

While attempting to get on a diabetic insulin supply trial, the initial examination revealed that the retinas in my eyes had grown blood vessels that were bleeding (diabetic retinopathy). I began receiving a series of laser surgeries over the next 15 years to attempt to seal the leaky vessels and to attempt to prevent any new vessel growth. This reduced my peripheral and night vision. In 1992, I developed an enlarged yet benign prostate gland and my kidneys began showing signs of deterioration. In 1993, I began experiencing some potency difficulties. In 1994, I began seeing a natural or homeopathic physician who, besides treating me with alternative medicine, advised me to increase my water intake. My intake of insulin was around 95 units of insulin daily.

In 1976, many immune system problems began developing. I graduated from high school in 1974 and went away to college. In 1976, I got a job as a mental health worker while going to school. I met my wife and while dating, working full time, and going to school part time, I developed "Infectious Mononucleosis." My wife and I were married in 1977, and I continued to struggle with many infections and illnesses as well as losing my job in 1978. In 1979, during one of my then frequent hospital stays, I was diagnosed with "mono" again! The doctors insisted that I shouldn't have it again and began consulting with specialists. I received an influenza vaccine and was discharged; only to be readmitted one day later with a fever of 106F°. I was undergoing many tests, however nothing much was showing up at that time. After many tests for severe abdominal pain, I was told that I grew a second spleen that was attached to my spleen and that the second one was also functioning. That year I was visiting someone, and drank unpasteurized milk and ended up in the hospital again with a bacterial infection of the intestinal tract. "Brucellosis and Proteus—ox-19" was the diagnosis and I was on yet more antibiotics.

During 1980 or 1981, I developed another case of "mono" and was admitted to the hospital again; diabetic control problems were a constant battle for me. An infectious disease specialist discovered that a number of special antibodies against foreign agents were also affected which the doctors suggested were related to the problems with my allergies and asthma, as well as my frequent infections.

The 1980s were filled with many hospitalizations, illnesses, job losses and stress-related problems. It was then that I was diagnosed with allergies to penicillin and tetracycline, began developing hypertension, was diagnosed with chronic fatigue syndrome, lymphoid hyperplasia (overstressed immune system), arthritis, bursitis, fibromyalgia, and gastroparesis or acid reflux problems, and bowel problems. I also developed a benign tumor on the left flank of my back. I developed a nodule on my thyroid area and was diagnosed with lead, cadmium and aluminum poisoning, which were also found in a landfill I lived near. I was overweight and developed sleep apnea. Tests showed that I stopped breathing over 300 times in a six-hour period and had "narcolepsy." I could fall asleep in a short period of time. I had surgery to attempt to correct the sleep apnea, and I wore a tracheotomy tube in my neck to help me breathe at night, and slept with a breathing machine to keep my airway open. During the 80s I still only drank a few glasses of water, yet consumed large amounts of coffee, saccharine and eventually NutraSweet. In 1987, I was declared "disabled"!

In 1992, at 36 years old, I looked and felt like I was in my late forties and felt worse than I looked. I began using natural supplements with vitamins, herbs, and other natural medical techniques. The natural doctor's advice was to increase my water consumption and decrease my caffeine intake as well. I had lost the feeling in my feet, was always tired and achy, depressed and had little hope.

I began to drink more water and reduced my caffeine intake somewhat and by 1995, I began to feel and look much better. Yet I was still only consuming a quart to a quart and a half daily, and not flushing all the caffeine out of my system nor was I using sea salt.

In September of 1995 that lump on my left flank turned red, and began itching and enlarging. My family physician removed it and sent it away for study. In October, I was diagnosed with cutaneous B-cell lymphoma. Twenty-six new tumors had grown on my back where there was one and I was sent to a major hospital where I was told that lymphatic cancer on the skin surface was rare and that not much research was done yet on it. I went for a gallium test and it revealed that my entire body surface glowed positive for cancer cells. The flank of my back was brighter white or "hyper-positive," as was the middle of my chest where two melanomas were previously removed. I was advised to receive localized radiation and as tumors appeared we would radiate them too or I could travel to Philadelphia and have my entire body surface radiated. They began to radiate my back, which began giving me third-degree burns. I refused total body radiation and midway through my radiation my homeopathic physician began using a natural cleansing therapy. The cancer specialist had advised me to try anything and to "pull out all the stops as well as to get my affairs in order." I increased my water consumption and took supplements and natural treatments.

In November of 1995, while traveling in search of an answer, I had to buy tires for my car. At the auto parts store where I was looking for tires, I was introduced to Bob Butts who exposed me to your *water cure program* and advised me to stick to it very seriously to get cured. I now began to seriously increase my water intake but was still leery of increasing salt intake due to the traditional medical contra-indications for its perceived high blood pressure problems. Later, I learned of the error of that thinking and began to increase my salt intake too. In March of "1996" I went for another gallium scan, which revealed that there was not a single sign of cancer glowing positive on my entire body. Doctors thought there was an error in the gallium scan, but my homeopath and I knew that I was healing. Drinking more water, reducing caffeine, and change in dietary habits, natural medicine and faith had brought me home. I acknowledge God's presence in me and remember the scripture, "I am the living waters." He called you and me "the salt of the earth," and tells us that we are "one in spirit."

Since then I've been constantly improving in my health. I no longer have two spleens, but one that is normal in size and function. Now I lick sea salt off my palm in the morning before my first glass of water and use salt liberally. I drink about 1.5 gallons of water a day and take some supplements as well as eating a lot of whole grains, and fresh fruits and vegetables. My waist used to be a size 40 and now is a size 36. I weighed 249 pounds, now I weigh 210 and have solid muscle mass. My complexion and appearance are those of a man in his early thirties and my potency of a man in his twenties. My ankles are no longer swollen and new pulses, yes new pulses have developed where once they were dead. I no longer take any medications for all those problems, whereas I used to be on at least 15 prescriptions at a time. My insulin needs are down from 95 units a day to 35–45 units a day. I no longer suffer with "chronic infections" or fatigue — I sleep 6–8 hours a day instead of 12–14. It is rare for me to take antibiotics, whereas I seemed to be constantly taking them before. I don't have allergies or asthma or gastroparesis (acid reflux) any more. I no longer suffer from arthritis, bursitis, or bowel problems. At the time of my last stress test, my doctor who is younger than I am told me that I was in better shape than he was. The high blood pressure is constantly improving. No more thyroid nodule, I sleep better and no more heavy metal toxicity. I have a new lease on life.

My prayers have been answered. God led me to a natural way to heal my body, my mind and my spirit. I am living a new life now with a balance of water, salt, minerals, supplements, good nutrition and continued improvements in my quality of life. I am truly blessed.

You have my permission to use this letter in any way you think will help spread the news of the medicinal value of water in medical treatment procedures.
Sincerely, Andrew J. Bauman, IV

💧   💧   💧

Asthma:

I have been plagued with asthma since I hit puberty at the age of 12. I have been hospitalized more times than I would like to count. On Wed. April 30, 2003, I was suffering terribly with breathing problems. I had not been able to sleep for 2 nights due to my breathing or lack thereof. So I called my Dr.'s office to see if I could get in to see the Dr. to get another Rx for steroids to calm the breathing down. He wasn't able to get me in so I was going to have to make do with my problem until Monday on my appointment. I thought to myself "I wonder what there is on the Net to help me?" So I typed in "How to stop an asthma attack" in my search bar and they returned several sites, yours was one of them.

I went to your site and read your info and tried it. IT WORKED ON THE 1st TRY! I have been trying everyday to increase my water intake and use the salt and water therapy to help my breathing. I am going to give up caffeine and try more of your suggestions.
I will keep you updated!!
Love Ya, V.

◊ ◊ ◊

Allergies; Asthma:

I have read your book and bought it for several people to read. I tell people to take the "water cure" every chance I get. I do want to say that I took Rx antihistamines for 20 years for severe allergies. Since I read your book, I haven't used any for over 3 years now and I am fine. Actually, taking an antihistamine or decongestant for a cold will trigger an allergic reaction for me. My two stepsons live with 5 cats and they formerly had asthma and severe allergies to cats—not anymore!! By the way, the best cure for poison ivy is WATER!
Thanks for your help.
Sincerely, L. G.

◊ ◊ ◊

Lupus:

Thank you for your book *Your Body's Many Cries for Water.* It was recommended to my husband and me so my husband bought it and after a brief look at it, decided it wasn't what we needed. He was about to return it, but I felt God wanted us to read it. I'm so glad we kept it.

I am very ill with lupus (SLE). I was starting to improve with an alternative treatment of low-dose pulsed antibiotic until my doctor treated me for an ulcer with Prilosec & Biaxin, plus a host of other drugs to treat the side effects of these drugs. I know he meant to help me, but he almost killed me with his medicines. It's been fifteen months and I'm barely starting to recover. How I wish I had known about the 12 cups of water to treat ulcers! The good news is that I am now off all medications (which always made me sicker anyway) for the first time in my life, I am eating a healthy diet (high protein, whole fresh foods and drinking plenty of water); I now have hope for a healthy body. I give the glory to my God who led me to your book, who also gave you the wisdom, and created this wonderful substance, water!

My husband suffers from psoriatic arthritis and our 13-year-old daughter was showing signs of rheumatic disease also. They have made the dietary changes including plenty of water and salt, and have been enjoying improved health also. All of us suffered terribly from allergies, but that has improved greatly!

What a joy to contemplate a future without innumerable doctors' visits and poisonous medicines. Thank you once again for making available this information in life-giving water. May God bless you.
Sincerely, R. L. S.

$\quad$ ♦ $\quad$ ♦ $\quad$ ♦

Note: I always leave the name of doctors, whose letters I use, in the text in case potential patients could contact them for help in their own case. After all, that is what doctors are about. Here is one such letter:

Shortness of Breath:

Once in a blue moon one comes across a really revolutionary book. It happens so seldom that those moments stand out as highlights. Your book *Your Body's Many Cries for Water* is such a book and moreover I finally know to whom I thank you for my recovery. This of course sounds strange so I will tell you.

In the summer of 1993 I was on vacation with my wife in Spain. On a hot day we went to the beach and paddled around in our rubber boat, that is to say, I paddled and my wife sat enjoying the water. Afterwards on the hottest moment of the day we climbed the steep rocky path back to our car and there and then my breath left me. I was 68 at that time so

I was not too astonished but the strange thing was, that my breath did not return. Ten days later we came back from that holiday and my breath was still somewhere on that rocky path. At least it did not come home with me. I resumed my practice and still I was out of breath. I had X rays taken as I had treated a woman with an open T.B., but showed nothing. When in the fall my breath still had not come back, I really began to worry. Then a good friend of mine, a doctor in New York gave me a telephone call and he asked me "You talk differently, what is the matter with your breath?" I told him about it and he said: "You did not drink enough water, you're the victim of bronchial constriction and this is caused by your body trying to save your water supplies." I had never heard that one before, but I took his advice and began to drink 8 glasses of water a day and in one week all my breathlessness had evaporated as if it had never been there. Since then I realized that in my youth I drank a lot of water but somewhere along the road I had lost the habit, so I began to drink more pure water (as my friend had stressed).

Everything went well until this winter. It was extremely cold in December, and I just stopped drinking all that cold water for a while. This happened to coincide with rather a strenuous dental repair, which was rather painful and suddenly I developed gastritis, with a tongue as white as snow. I suddenly remembered that my N.Y. friend had told me that another pathway the body chose to stop losing water was by closing the pylorus. I straight away started taking 8 glasses of water again (happily the cold had lessened considerably) and within four days my stomach was healed, much to the surprise of a young colleague who worked with me at that moment and who never had heard of a gastritis healing so fast.

You asked for corroborating evidence, so this is why I send you this lengthy letter. I have been a medical practitioner for 27 years and after that (since 1981) I left general practice and now I am a consultant on allergy, food and chemical intolerances and holistic treatment of cancer. I have already used the water treatment for asthma in my extensive children's practice (half of my patients are under ten years old) and I definitely see results. So I can say from personal experience, both on myself and in my practice, that I can affirm what you have found. I will try to get your book printed in the Netherlands.

If ever you find time to write me back: There is a furious discussion going on in my doctors' group. One half says: No water in cancer patients, only fruit and vegetable juices. I belong to those who are saying: lots of pure water! I know that you will agree with me, but it would be nice if you affirm my knowledge. Another thing is, you mention bulimia as one of the illnesses related to dehydration, but what about anorexia nervosa? Finally, eczema is not only on the increase, but it becomes more and more resistant to anti-allergic measures (which in my practice means finding out the offending foods and chemical substances, etc.). Is that possibly a case of dehydration too? The American way of life (cola, etc.) becomes more popular all the time in my country.

I understand fully when you find no time to write me back, but in any case, I want to thank you for having written your wonderful book. You are a worthy representative of one of the oldest civilizations in the world. With many good wishes,
Yours sincerely,
Hans C. Moolenburgh

PS: I am convinced that my New York friend must have heard about your work and so could help me straight away. Did not ask him at the time how he came by this knowledge.

I would never have suspected people in a wet country like ours to suffer from dehydration. It never entered my mind.

◆   ◆   ◆

Dry Cough; Asthma; Bronchitis:

I am writing to thank you for the cure I got from chronic bronchitis, asthma and a chronic cough with water and salt.

Sir Harold Klemp, Living ECK Master, told us about your book, *Your Body's Many Cries for Water* at an ECKANKAR seminar.

I had this cough for many years and several doctors tried to "cure" me of it with many drugs. I could clear a room when I coughed; people looked at me like I had the plague.

My present doctor, a lung specialist, gave up on it. "I'd sure like to get rid of that cough," he'd say. But he could not. After I read your book, I drank (3) 8 oz glasses of water every morning and took a pinch of salt, cough up some phlegm and the cough is gone. No more carrying an inhaler everywhere I go. No more asthma attacks. I drink at least eight glasses of water a day now. I carry it everywhere I go.

I've given several of the books away and told others about it. Several people I know are using the techniques in the book.

Thank you again. This book can save lives.
Sincerely, E. S.

Joint Flexibility; Sinus Problems:

This letter has a two-fold purpose: (1) to thank you and tell you how your research has positively affected my life and (2) to ask your permission to photocopy specific pages of your books so that people will know who, what, where and how to obtain additional information and materials on this subject.

My friend Esther has been prodding me to write to you for almost a year since discovering your book and subsequently using the information you discovered and researched. Forgive me for taking so long to write and thank you for the health benefits I have received from drinking adequate amounts of pure water every day as a result of finding out the role water plays in the human body.

The benefits I received immediately are:

- I stopped using antihistamines
- My skin is no longer dry
- My sinus problems so far are history
- My finger joints are more flexible (I use a computer every day for my job)
- My energy level has increased; and last but not least,
- I have more clarity of mind and seem to think and remember things better (I'll stop here as I could go on and on).

Though I did not show my appreciation immediately by writing to inform you of these blessings, I did immediately begin to share this information and tell anybody who would listen.

As a result of the blessings I have received, I feel God would have me share this as so many people are suffering when water would in many cases take care of the condition. That is why I'm in the process of developing a ministry to help individuals improve their daily lives by addressing areas that affect us mentally, physically, and spiritually. Our relationship with "water" will be the first topic presented.

Here is where I am asking your permission to copy the cover of your book, *Your Body's Many Cries for Water*, and pages 1, 2, 46, & 48 of your book, *Water: Rx for a Healthier Pain-Free Life*, so that as I stated in the beginning, people will know how to obtain additional information and materials on this subject.
Cordially, K. M. D.

Acid Reflux; Asthma:

Just a brief message to let you know that after just 7 days on 2 liters of water per day plus a half teaspoonful of salt I have experienced a dramatic improvement in my stomach problems—peptic ulcer, heartburn and reflux. Last night I was able to eat a late meal and not have to worry about throwing up; I am still a little gassy but do not have heartburn any more. I think my asthma has also improved. I will provide a more detailed report in about four weeks. Thank you so much for sharing your wonderful health discoveries with me and the rest of the world.

I have tried your cure, and the missing ingredient for me anyway was salt. I was not consuming very much salt. In the olden days, the people used to preserve things with salt. Now everything is salt free; I even see salt-free salt. It could be that people are depleted of salt. My asthma did not start till 5 years after being married to my wife, who is a very healthy eater and consequently, I have been getting the salt I used to. I found that 1.5 tsp. of salt taken per day seems to help my asthma so far with the water of course.

Thank you for this amazing discovery, I also take ju-jitsu class and for the past 3 years have been waiting to be able to take a class without the puffer. Maybe the salt will do this. I tell people at work about this (I work in a hospital), but am perceived as somewhat of an oddity for saying that I am taking salt.
Sincerely, N. B.

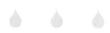

**Acne; Sinus Infection;
Constipation:**

I thought you might be interested to know what water drinking has done for me. It has eliminated my acne, my serious constipation problem, my sinus infections, my tonsil infections; and I have not succumbed to any colds or flu since I started drinking more water. I now realize people are sick because they aren't drinking enough water or they are eating too much sugar. I have never felt better or looked better in my whole life and I'm 43 years old. It is such a shame that I didn't realize this 25 years ago. I now drink 3 quarts. of warm water a day, one quart before breakfast. Who knows how much disease could be prevented if this simple remedy alone was followed. Your book is fantastic, thanks for educating the public on this most necessary and vital subject.
Sincerely, Mrs. Connie Allen, R.N.B.S.

Allergies; Asthma:

Since I was an infant, I had been plagued with chronic allergic and environmental asthma. I am 35 years old, and up until 2 years ago when my father sent me a copy of your wonderful book on water, I was completely dependent on bronchodilators.

As a child I took liquid Marax, as a teenager I took oral theophylline, and as an adult I was on 3 combinations of inhaled steroids and B-agonist bronchodilators (prednisone & Ventolin). I was worn out from fighting for breath, and nervous and shaky from the medicines' side effects.

Then 2 years ago, I began following the recommendations in your wonderful book. I have not only been asthma free for over 2 years now, but am also able to go running without medication, as I do 3–4 times a week.

You have given my life back to me. Bless you and your work.
Sincerely, C. C. B.

💧   💧   💧

Nephrosis; Allergies; Cold Hands and Feet; Mental Fog:

I suffered from childhood nephrosis for more than 10 years. (Adrenal hormones signal kidneys to retain salt and spill protein in urine; edema.) As an adult I suffered from allergies. I started drinking large amounts (1–2 gallons) of water daily about 20 years ago. This helped, but I still suffered from allergies and occasional bouts of edema during long gray winters when outside activity was limited. Cold hands and feet, dull aches and pains were common, mental acuity was slow. Summers were different when I felt energetic and mentally clear. My summer diet included more salt. Years of searching modern medical and alternative health information left me puzzled. Then I discovered your work. I increased my salt intake to recommended levels and it all went away. Most significant: improved mental clarity, edema gone, dull muscle aches gone, hands and feet now warm, no allergies or nasal congestion. Increased energy, balanced urination throughout the day and I sleep better. It is easier to fall asleep. I awake more refreshed. Sugar cravings are a thing of the past. Nervous energy transformed into productive energy. My memory improved.

I'm lucky that the prednisone and salt-free diet as a child didn't kill me. I suspect the hospitalization treatment, which included IVs, were the real cure. I get healthier every year and many cannot believe my age.

Thanks for revealing such simple, wonderful information. I see your work as a part of the "Christ Consciousness" being revealed to help humanity. Metaphysically, water is a step-down transducer of high-dimensional spiritual energy into the physical plane. We get the Holy Spirit more efficiently when we are hydrated. It is one of the great esoteric secrets.

God Bless You! F. A. R.

         ◊   ◊   ◊

Note: The following two letters are from another medical doctor, whose son had asthma and is now cured. The second letter is an update. Dr. Christopher practices family medicine in the Baltimore area and now understands water as a medication if, and when any of my readers would like to visit her at her office. *Please, please avoid curiosity calls.* The word *coryza* used in the letter means "infection of the upper respiratory tract."

Allergic Rhinitis; Asthma:

Reference: Jeremy Christopher

I am writing to thank you for your kind assistance in treating Jeremy's allergies. As you know Jeremy is my eight-year-old son who suffered for the last 3–4 years with severe allergy symptoms related to allergic rhinitis and asthma.

More recently, he has had significant coryza and coughing which is associated with his asthma. On about the 28th of April 1995, we began a program of re-hydration involving his drinking two cups of water before food or exercise and excluding all other fluids. In addition, he consumes a half-teaspoon of salt, which is added to his food to offset the increased water intake.

Within 3–4 days he showed dramatic improvement, he no longer had severe and excessive mucus production, his coughing had virtually stopped and his sneezing and other allergy symptoms were totally gone. Therefore we discontinued his Benadryl and albuterol and continued his hydration program.

Jeremy has been following this program now for approximately four and a half weeks, spending almost four weeks off his medication and is doing quite well. Not only have his symptoms cleared subjectively, but also in terms of objective findings, his peak flow volumes have been within normal range. His constant medication-induced drowsiness has disappeared and as a result he is more alert, and his school grades have improved.

Therefore I want to emphasize how effective this treatment has been for Jeremy and I wish you well in sharing this cost effective and very efficacious program with others.

Once again Dr. Batmanghelidj, I thank you for advising me on the new treatment program of Jeremy's allergies and asthma.
Very truly yours, Cheryl Brown-Christopher, M.D.

Re: Jeremy Christopher—UPDATE

Once again, I am writing to thank you and update you on the results from your precious advice regarding water intake and allergies for my son, Jeremy. As you may recall, four years ago, Jeremy at the age of eight, had severe symptoms of allergic rhinitis, including runny eyes, continuous sneezing, coughing and reduced mental concentration. He additionally had been diagnosed with asthma. Inhalers and antihistamines provided minimal benefit, and plans were in progress to begin desensitization injections (allergy shots). Fortunately, during this period of time, we met and you advised me to begin Jeremy on your protocol of drinking 6–8 glasses of water daily along with 1/2 teaspoon of salt per day. Within two weeks, Jeremy's symptoms had completely resolved and his peak flow meter readings increased over 50%. In essence, Jeremy's lung volume readings became normal and his hay fever cleared without medication!!

Jeremy is now a twelve-year-old, upcoming seventh grader who has never taken allergy shots and is doing well after four years of following the "Batman water protocol." To be candid Dr. Batmanghelidj, my son will periodically drink sodas or juices and experience very short-lived flare-ups of sneezing when exposed to ragweed, pollen or dust concurrently with drinking these beverages. Fortunately, the symptoms clear very rapidly with his ingesting two glasses of water and 1/2 teaspoon of salt or salty foods.

My husband and I continue to monitor Jeremy's peak flow meter readings only sporadically now, as he has been asymptomatic with respect to asthma for four years and his readings are always normal. I have been so impressed with these results, Dr. Batmanghelidj, that I advise every patient in my orthopedic medicine and family practice to follow your protocol. I have seen remarkable improvements in patients with allergies including asthma, attention deficit disorder, diabetes, back pain, arthritis, hypertension, and many other chronic illnesses that follow your protocol.

Dr. Batman, in my opinion, Jeremy is cured of asthma and allergic rhinitis as a result of your outstanding research on the benefits of water. This breakthrough approach to allergies and other chronic diseases is effective, convenient, and affordable to all. I am deeply grateful to you as both a mother and a physician. May God bless you in your continued efforts to spread the word to all.
Sincerely, Cheryl Brown-Christopher, M.D.
Diplomate, AAPM, FAAFP

Weight Loss; Asthma:
Allergies; Bronchitis; Cravings for Alcohol;
Acne; Arthritis:

For some time now, I have been trying to write to you to inform you of my progress using your system of the "Water Cure." As you know, I seriously started your program back in 1997.

I lost 30 pounds in 31 days, lost all symptoms of my 19 years of asthma, allergies and bronchitis as well as lost all desires for alcohol. I remember people telling me how my skin "glowed" which was in itself a miracle because I had such bad acne not only on my face, but also on my shoulders, back and arms. On top of all that, I had arthritis on my hands. It was especially hard to decorate cakes and cookies, which I did professionally, because of the pain. I no longer have that problem either.

Now let me do a breakdown. I weighed approx. 192 pounds and I am 5'4" tall, or shall I say that is how short I am. I am now down to and remaining steady at 160 (give or take a few pounds because of the holidays). I can now fit into clothes I never was able to get in but I knew I would one day. You can't imagine how great it feels to have my kids and others call me "skinny" instead of the Crisco Kid—fat in the can! But the best feeling is when Bob holds me and his arms fit all around me now and then some.

When I first met you, I had allergies that were so bad that my eyes would swell up each and every morning. They itched so unbearably that I became addicted to an eye cream that the doctors has given me. Instead of drinking the iced tea, you told me to put it on my eyes and it worked. I stopped drinking all caffeine at that point but I was not able to give up the beer at that time. That came later. I had bronchitis twice a year, which was devastating. I could count on having an attack when the seasons changed from summer to fall and winter into spring. I'm sure my doctor has probably given me up for dead, because I have not had to call him in years for the antibiotic and cough medicine. Just this past Thanksgiving, someone asked me if I were using a special lotion for my face because I looked younger.

With all the problems I "had" in the past, I know that it is difficult to explain to someone that the simplicity of it all is hydration as well as nutrition, but it is.

I will be eternally grateful for your discovery and all your help Dr. Batman. May God be with us all in spreading this discovery.
Connie Giblin

Note: I did not edit Connie's name because like me, she lives for the time that the information on water could spread to all parts of the globe.

Lupus; Muscle and Joint Pains:

I would like to express my grateful appreciation of your book *Your Body's Many Cries for Water*. I first read this in March this year, by loan from a friend, and was immediately convinced of your paradigm.

So many give advice of what is needed for specific problems but do not explain why. I need to know the reason of things. Your reasoning, with such applied science, gave me impetus to buy this book for myself together with the *ABC of Asthma, Allergies and Lupus*, and *How to Deal with Back Pain*. (Tagman Press was very prompt and courteous in dealing with this.) My wife suffers from bronchial asthma and my particular problem is lupus. After studying your books carefully, and making an extract for myself of the salient practical points, my wife and I have been drinking only water, 8 glasses and a little extra salt each day since March.

The benefits I have noticed with my lupus (S.L.E.) are a dramatic improvement in my energy level (very little fatigue), which was always a big problem; joint and muscle pains have almost disappeared. (I should say that I still take 71/2 mg of prednisolone daily which masks things a bit), muscle and skin tone have also improved a lot.

Like you, I am 71, and in my youth used to play a lot of tennis, some-times up to 4–5 hrs. When I think back I drank very little during these times. At about 28 I developed problems in both shoulders, such pain that I could only serve under-arm, eventually having to give up playing. The consultant I saw at the time injected as far as I can remember about 1 milli-liter of cortisone into each shoulder muscle. From that time on in my life I developed extreme eczema, joint pains which con-tinued a long time with many varied treatments sought, alleviated to a certain degree. Then in 1984 diagnosed with polymyalgia rheumatica and finally about 1996 S.L.E. lupus. Considering your observations, research and findings, I sense that my case is typical of a lot of people's imbalance through years of unintentional drought, not giving the nec-essary requirements of a true solute balance. It certainly explains to me why I became so underweight and drained of energy.

Thank you for your great effort to place this information before us, the general public.

With regard to my wife's asthma, she had a particularly bad time at the beginning of this year (Jan/Feb), confined to bed for about 6 weeks, four or five courses of antibiotic, and interestingly could only drink water. She did not want any other beverages. Her main eating was light salad meals, and her improvement was gradual to the middle of February when she was clear of coughing up mucus. She had lost a lot of weight but did begin to put some on. This was an added incentive for me to obtain your books. By the time I studied your books and then was applying the water treatment (end of March) her cough had returned somewhat. Her clearance of the mucus every morning and during the day is easier than before, but seems so deep in the lungs that it takes a lot of effort.

At 68, I recognize that a lifelong sufferer may not obtain a full reversal, but if you have a moment for advice perhaps I could ask your help with a question. On the rule of thumb you give (1/2 ounce of water to every 1 lb of weight) my wife should have 3 pints of water a day. (Her weight is 120 lbs). My question is, do you think that increasing the salt would be advisable, and possibly the amount of water to assist her constant congestion? Her skin texture and elasticity has improved considerably with good color in her cheeks. She has no other medical problems, good heart, kidneys, and blood pressure. Her normal medication is a Ventolin Diskhaler and Flixotide Diskhaler, but with a recent addition by her doctor of an inhaler salmeterol 25. I would appreciate your advice to my question, and any help you may be able to give for her asthma.

I hope, Dr. Batmanghelidj your tour goes well in this country, and once again many thanks for your determined persistence in presenting your findings to a willing public against reluctant professionals.
With kind regards, D. R.

Note: I included this letter and their question to explain that salt is a vital element to health and well-being of the body. When you drink water in the quantities that your body needs, you will gradually wash out some of the essential minerals that are dissolved in the body fluids. You need to constantly replace that which you lose. Sea salt is a good source of some of these minerals. However, sea salt does not contain enough iodine to keep your thyroid gland healthy. You need to make sure your supplements contain iodine. Salt is vital for the normal physiology of your lungs.

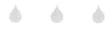

Note: The next two letters are from Jose A. Rivera, M.D. He was the associate professor of medicine at the Capital University of Integrative Medicine in Washington, D.C. He now practices complementary medicine in South Carolina.

Allergies to Cat; Asthma:

Since my letter of 1-6-95, I have been asthma free for approximately 4 years since initially being introduced to your prescription for health in taking water and salt as preventive measures that also cured my asthma attacks. Remembering to watch for signs of stress and fatigue, which can induce bronchial constriction for water preservation and rationing. This is very important since it is during these times that one is unaware of what is really happening physiologically.

Listening to one's own body can enable one to prevent what was once a common occurrence, bronchial constriction that later leads to asthma. It is through these simple directions of hydrating the body with water and regulating the salt levels that one can begin to prevent and cure asthma and heal a body in need of better hydration.

Your prescription for health is certainly a constant reminder to recovering asthmatics.

Thank you for your attention and constant help.
Sincerely, Jose A. Rivera, M.D.

Enclosed is a summary of some patients who have been treated with water as part of their therapeutic treatment.

Patient #1 Asthma:

12-year-old white male with history of asthma (non-exertional). Patient has been seen by pediatrician and was put on Proventil inhaler. Patient's mother was given misinformation by pediatrician who stated that when a crisis arose to take as many puffs of Proventil until asthma subsides. Because of this misinformation, when patient had next crisis the mother gave the patient 6 puffs of Proventil with no amelioration but exacerbation of the symptoms of wheezing, chest tightness, light-headedness and restlessness. The patient was able to lie down but continued to wheeze extensively. The mother gave us a call around 10:30 P.M. with the complaint of wheezing and chest tightness of her son. Immediately we told her to give her son two 8 oz. glasses of water and a pinch of salt on his tongue. We then told her to call us back in 5 minutes for further instructions. To our surprise her son stopped wheezing and his chest tightness had decreased. He was then able to lie down and sleep. The patient has been instructed to continue to drink water and use salt if another attack occurred. The mother has been made aware that if other medications are needed, to use them as instructed.

Patient #2 Hypertension; Edema:

67-year-old white female with H/O myocardial infarction, stroke, diabetic retinopathy, hypertension. This patient was seen initially because of her diabetic retinopathy. The patient's above past medical history was under control but we felt that she needed to change some of her fluid intake modality due to occasional hypertension and unilateral pedal edema. The patient was encouraged to drink two 8 oz. glasses of water before each meal and to cut coffee and other sugar-free drinks from her diet. Within a few days, the patient observed that she was urinating much better and that her pressure had begun to stabilize. She also stated that she had begun to feel much better and that her leg swelling had diminished noticeably. The patient continues to supplement water as part of her normal daily diet.

Our initial observation has been with compliance from all our patients. It is a common practice to tell all patients to eliminate coffee, soft drinks and other beverages and substitute with water. This shift in thinking has been the major obstacle, but we are encouraged when a patient who has felt the need to comply comes with good news of amelioration of symptoms.

We hope that we can continue to give you more reports on our progress as they arrive.

Thank you for your attention.
Sincerely, Jose A. Rivera M.D.

$\bullet$ $\bullet$ $\bullet$

Lupus; Acne:

I am writing to thank you for the discoveries you have made, and the results you have published in *ABC of Asthma, Allergies and Lupus*. My 15-yr-old daughter is a busy and healthy (or so I thought) teenager who lifeguarded at a country club pool during the summer.

She became severely ill while she was away at an out-of-town cheerleading camp where the temperature in the field house was 108 degrees Fahrenheit. By the time she got home, she was very feverish, had blood red urine, and she said it hurt when she breathed. Her fever climbed as high as 105 for several hours. When I took her to the doctor, they tested her four times for mononucleosis and strep throat, because she also had large white spots in the back of her throat, which were misdiagnosed as an infection or virus. They also tested her for Hepatitis A, B, and C, all of which came up negative.

Realizing that my daughter was in a crisis that was not being answered by the medical community, I took myself to the library to search for any information that might help her. Although the doctors had disagreed with me, and told me not to label my daughter with such a debilitating and degenerative disease, I noticed that many of her symptoms matched those that my medical guide labeled lupus. She had had Raynaud's syndrome since childhood, and with this latest illness developed pain in the chest when breathing (the doctor had ruled out pneumonia), red urine, headache, tiredness and fatigue, and also the malar flush, plus fever over 100 degrees. Another symptom that mystified the doctors is that her white blood count was extremely low.

I decided I must find out more about lupus and any known causes. At that time, the only book at the library on the topic was *The ABC of Asthma, Allergies, and Lupus.* Within minutes of opening your book, I realized that my daughter was suffering from severe, chronic dehydration and lack of salt in her body. She has never cared for salty foods, although we had noticed that she would start laughing and get a "natural high" from eating Ramen noodles, her one salty source. We immediately urged her to drink and take salt to replenish her body of the fluids she had lost, not only at the cheer camp, but over the summer as a lifeguard, and even during the prior school year where her one beverage of the day was a Diet Coke. Although I had been in the habit of drinking several small glasses of water per day, I didn't realize that my daughter's only fluid intake besides the Diet Coke had been a small glass of orange juice for breakfast, and a glass of milk at dinner.

Within days she was so much better, it was wonderful to see. The nurse who drew her blood on Thursday was the same one who had drawn her blood on Monday before I checked out your book. She had made no comment on Monday, but on Thursday she said the blood was "leaping from her veins," while it had been only "dribbling" out on Monday. Within days every one of Jenny's symptoms disappeared and her blood tests returned to normal.

Jenny appears to have completely returned to good health. We have also increased her protein intake, as she was only eating minimal amounts. When Jenny was so ill, the doctor ordered her to stop taking her acne medication, and what we discovered is that, since Jenny has been drinking much more water, she has no need to resume taking the antibiotics. Her face is almost completely clear with no medication at all.

Increasing our water and salt intake has helped each member of our family. My athletic son had suffered from severe back pain and headaches. The back pain has been eliminated and his headaches are much less frequent and much less intense. My headaches have been reduced and my outlook is so much better. My youngest daughter has noticed a marked reduction in allergy and sinus problems since she has followed your guidelines for water and salt. Even my husband has noticed it is easier to lose weight when you are getting adequate water and salt.

Thank you for your research and work in this field. You may have saved my daughter from severe illness or even death. I see the connection of many conditions, some acute, some chronic, most tied to the water/salt balance in us. Thank you again.

I have since purchased my own copies of *Your Body's Many Cries for Water* and *The ABC of Asthma, Allergies, and Lupus*. I have referred so many of my friends and family to your books and everybody knows somebody who can be helped by this information. I am also eagerly awaiting *The ABC of Cancer and Depression*.
Sincerely, M. L.

Author's Note:

I was browsing the Internet to see how many Web sites have become engaged in the dissemination of information on the medicinal properties of water, when I came across the article that is published below. I wrote to the author, and asked for permission to share his experience with the readers of this book. He graciously wrote me the following message and let me share his personal discovery of the pain-relieving property of water with you. The letter and the article come to you as their author wrote them.

Dr. Batmanghelidj,

You have been my hero for a long time. I have told people that you are the undisputed leader in the world on the harmful effects of dehydration and the human need for water. Of course you may use my story in your new book. The story is from my book *Pain Free for Life*. It was just published this year. There are 80,000 copies in print. In the book I tell about you Dr. Batmanghelidj in several places. I would be honored for you to use my story.
Darrell Stoddard, Founder—Pain Research Institute

It Is Better to Wet Your Pants
than Live with Chronic Pain

"The extra water you drink when you take a pill

does more good than the pill"

Darrell J. Stoddard, Copyright 1998

I couldn't walk across the floor for a hundred dollars a step when I first got up in the morning. My left ankle that I injured hurt so bad that I would nearly pass out if I put weight on it. Then after hopping around on one foot for a while I was able to hobble through the day. The thing that made my injury even more distressing is that I am a pain specialist who had stopped the pain in more than 9000 patients and I couldn't help myself.

My regular morning runs that I had been doing faithfully for 26 years came to an end. The goal of running like my acquaintance Larry Lewis (who at 103 years of age ran six miles every morning before going to work) was now impossible.

I had my foot X-rayed. There were no fractures or broken bones. I tried my own treatments, Bioelectric and Auricular Therapy. It did nothing for the pain. I had orthotics made, had my ankle taped, did all of the exercises given to me by a podiatrist, injected my foot with vitamin B-6 and B-12, injected all of the trigger points with procaine. I took vitamins and minerals of all kinds, tried glucosamine sulfate, glucosamine hydrochloride, phenylalanine, blue-green algae, cod-liver oil, flaxseed oil and non-fat yogurt, pygnoginal, etc.

When all of the natural stuff failed, I tried aspirin, Tylenol and a number of non-steroidal anti-inflammatory drugs. Some of these made the pain a little more bearable but when I stopped taking them the pain came back with a vengeance. I was obviously just masking the pain and making myself vulnerable for further injury. For nine months I tried everything ever heard of for pain short of narcotics. By now I was getting desperate. My goal and dream of running till I was 100 years old was now just that, only a dream. People were coming to me from all over the world to stop their pain and I couldn't help myself.

I read the book *Your Body's Many Cries for Water* by F. Batmanghelidj, M.D. that I highly recommend. (Available from *amazon.com*. Click on the link and type in book title to learn about purchase.) I started drinking more water, or at least thought I was, but I wasn't consistent enough to help and my pain continued.

A patient of mine who was an engineer developed a water softener/purification system that used potassium chloride instead of sodium chloride. They came to our house to test the water and do a demonstration. The demonstration included filling a bowl full of water and showing how much chlorine was in it. I then was instructed to immerse my hand in the water and stir it for five minutes. After stirring the water, it was again tested and the chlorine was all gone. I was told that the chlorine was absorbed by my hand and this is the reason I needed a whole house water conditioning system, not just the drinking water—because the chlorine which is a toxic poison would be absorbed into the body while taking a shower or a bath.

I told Dr. Remington with whom I work about the demonstration and he said, "Some of the chlorine may have been absorbed but most of it evaporated. That is why," he said, "you have to keep putting chlorine in a swimming pool, because it evaporates." He then added, "If you want to solve that problem, let your drinking water sit overnight without a lid on it and all of the chlorine will evaporate."

I started doing this and at the end of the day I could see how much water I did not drink. This routine reminded me to consistently drink more water. *Lo and behold the painful foot that stopped me from running and crippled me for nine months got better.*

Now each morning I can again go running like I did before the injury. Through the experience, I learned as much about stopping pain as I did in a lifetime of study. Dr. Batmanghelidj is right, when we are in pain our bodies are "crying for water." Besides having the pain in my foot go away, another interesting change came into my life, several times a day I have to run for the bathroom like a little child, something I haven't done for more than fifty years. One of these days I'm not going to make it, but it will be worth it.

I knew better. One of my father's favorite sayings was, "The *extra* water you drink when you take a pill does you more good than the pill."

Asthma/Blindness:
Can there be a connection?

I have had asthma for three years and have been treated by an allergist and doctor. Each time I would get a cold (which was frequently), I would also get this horrible cough. Other than the colds and asthma I was perfectly healthy.

Last year after having a cold and cough I developed optic neuritis in my left eye, which left me with only 20% vision in that eye. This year after having a cold and terrible cough again, I developed optic neuritis in my right eye. You cannot imagine the despair I experienced when this happened because I had been to the best eye hospitals in the East and had been told they could not find a reason for this optic neuritis (they put me through every test imaginable) and they had no cure or operation or any kind of hope for me.

My doctors here treated me with steroids and saved my sight in my right eye. At the same time I was told about the "Water Cure" for asthma and grabbed at this because it was the only real lifeline I had left. (You have to picture a widow, living alone, not being able to drive or take care of her home, or go to work without begging for help from family and friends. I really thought my life was over.) Immediately I began drinking 64 oz. of water every day and in two days I stopped coughing and have not coughed for five months now or even had a cold, which is a miracle for me.

I am now able to drive, work, cut grass, shovel snow and go for walks and except for the damage done to my left eye, lead a perfectly healthy normal life. I do see a slight improvement in my eyes and I am hoping that if I can stay cough free for a while, I may get more sight back.

We all think because we drink a lot of coffee, tea, soda or juice we are getting all the fluids we need, but we don't realize that most of these drinks can dehydrate your body. Water is the most inexpensive, non-invasive, healthy thing we can do for ourselves.
Sincerely, S. P.

Asthma; Allergies to Milk and Pollen;
Sleep; Weight Loss:

One year ago, April 1999, we read the book, *Your Body's Many Cries for Water*, available at www.watercure.com. We had been hoping for this kind of miracle, which would allow our family, and especially our 11-year-old asthmatic child, to live a normal life, so we decided to try it. What did we have to lose? Even if 1/10 of what was claimed was effective in our case it would still be a great improvement, and it wouldn't cost much.

Within days, several results were obvious, especially the asthma and its related problems. Over the last year, we have gone from almost weekly visits to the doctor for someone in the family, plus hundreds of dollars in medicines, to virtually none. Below is a list of changes (sometimes dramatic) that we have noticed in our family's health. These have come from the simple change to drinking water as almost our only beverage, and drinking it in abundance.

- All wounds heal much faster
- Strength that had been lost has returned to ankles and wrists
- Allergies to both milk and pollens have disappeared
- Asthma is gone—no more medication, decongestants, antihistamines or inhalers
- Sore ribs from hard bed gone—previously needed a special pad
- Shinier hair with much more body
- Impetigo gone
- Smoother skin, with less wrinkling on face and elbows now rarely requiring lotion
- Dark, healthy skin on Black children, with little lotion
- 11-year-old lost 10 excess pounds
- No more ear infections
- Sleep great after 20 years of insomnia
- Good appetite increase in child with asthma
- School grades from D– to A/Bs for child with asthma
- No more motion sickness
- No more antibiotics for bronchial problems related to asthma
- Much more pep and energy
- Arthritis in fingers gone

It has taken a while for the children to get used to the new program, and getting them to continue to drink enough water daily is a challenge. Several of us have added significant salt to our diet to prevent headaches, control eye tearing and promote sleep. We have not been successful in using water drinking to automatically lose excess weight, but in all other areas, we are fully satisfied. Except for weight loss, all the book's claims that we were able to verify have been completely confirmed in our lives.

We would be delighted to talk to anyone who might be interested about our experiences. We fully support any effort to encourage the medical, pharmaceutical and beverage industries to recognize the essential nature of water drinking to the human body and to discontinue their commercialized profit-driven assault on our health.
Thank you, C. S. H.

Sinus Infection:

The very highest of accolades and kudos to you for authoring *Your Body's Many Cries for Water*. A friend, who resides here and has recently written you advising the numerous benefits from following your recommended regimen of water consumption, gave your book to me. He experienced amazingly rapid results from a chronic sinus condition that had plagued him from youth.

Now it's my turn to similarly attest to the efficacy of your program. Because of the plethora of information advocating deletion of all salt from your diet, I had virtually eliminated salt, except for the small amount ingested from normal cooking. I have experienced a lifetime of catarrhal congestion at intermittent intervals, and just expected it to be perpetual. Because of your admonition to include salt purposely in reasonably small amounts, I decided to try it, with astounding results!! Not even a sniffle, and I intend to adhere to this henceforth. As well, your book precipitated an immediate paradigm metamorphosis in the amounts of water-consumed daily.

Thank you for this information and for all that you're doing to spread the word.
Sincerely yours, J. R. P.

Asthma; Persistent Cough:

I suffered from asthma as a small child, which eventually subsided. However I continued to have debilitating bouts of bronchitis every winter of my life. I cannot remember a single year when I did not have a persistent, hacking cough, starting in the fall and continuing through March. One time this coughing was so violent that I had to be taken to the ER. Other times I actually pulled muscles and in one case injured a rib from repeated and violent coughing. Doctors kept prescribing antibiotics, but they had absolutely no effect on the problem, and in fact created other symptoms that just made things worse.

This October, I was really dreading what I knew would be six long months of suffering for me and my husband (who is kept awake nights listening to me cough). In my morning contemplation (my religion's form of prayer), I asked to be shown a solution to my problem. Immediately, I heard the word "water," and I knew at once that drinking more water would somehow help me, though I wasn't sure how.

I was never much of a water drinker, so I began to drink more water; I increased my intake to the usual 6–8 glasses a day that doctors usually advise. Amazingly, I had no signs of the bronchitis. But somehow I doubted that the inner guidance I had received was accurate. I began to doubt the correlation between my increased water intake and my improved health. I guess the mind is always looking for facts and figures to back up what the part of us that is divine already knows. In any case, just as my period of doubting began, someone at work told me about your book and I ordered it. Your book was the "proof" I was looking for!! Your explanation of how dehydration leads to asthma and bronchitis was crystal clear to me, and gave me the renewed determination to keep drinking more water. I also added the salt to my diet.

I do not follow your regimen as completely as I would like to. But when I begin slipping, I notice a little congestion in my chest, and I again become attentive to my water intake. I am amazed to report that I have made it through the first winter of my life without any bronchitis, and without the persistent, hacking cough that has troubled me every year of my life.

I am incredibly grateful for your work and hope you are able to distribute this information in a more global way, as I feel much suffering could be alleviated and many misspent medical dollars saved if only people understood the significance of water to the body's functioning.
In heartfelt gratitude, R. S.

Allergies; Bronchitis; Watery Eyes; Hiatal Hernia:

I received your tapes and your books and I have been drinking 64 oz of water each day now for 8 days now. I have always been one to drink a lot of water, more than any of my family or friends. I often wondered how they could go forever without water. But I still did not drink enough I guess. Since I have started drinking as you directed I have felt so much better. I have used Celtic salt for quite some time now, I've never used store-bought salt; but Celtic salt is wonderful, I sent to North Carolina for it. I have gotten my daughter and my sister to start drinking more water and my other sister in Arizona is going to start drinking water too.

I had a terrible bronchial cough, watery eyes, allergies, achy bones and joints and a little overweight. I have lost five pounds, eyes do not water as much, my bones and joints don't ache, and I am almost over my hiatal hernia or acid reflux, whichever it was. I have almost lost my craving for sweets, and I can stand on one foot to put on my slacks, which before I had to sit on the bed to do. My hair is looking better; the liver spots are beginning to disappear.

I think your knowledge about drinking water is the most important medical information that has come along in years and years and I believe in what you're saying. Most of the medical profession and the drug companies and scientists are looking for a way to put money in their pocket, that's why really simple and useful things hold no interest for them. If I sound bitter, I'm not, just discouraged and disappointed with a profession that took an oath and broke it. There are some good ones, thanks to them we have progressed as far as we have in the business of healing. I praise God for men like you and others who have really worked for the good of others.
Sincerely, A. S.

Asthma:

I am writing to share my situations with you and offer information that could be helpful to you and those you love and care for.

Three weeks ago my 10-year-old son Aaron was diagnosed with allergies (to almost everything but food) and asthma. He had suffered most of the fall and winter with nasal congestion, coughing and a constant need to clear his throat. When these symptoms did not respond to traditional treatments, our pediatrician referred us to an allergy specialist. The allergist prescribed 5 different medications/inhalers to use three times per day and gave us a booklet on how we needed to change our lives and our environment. After this appt., my very active, happy child was upset, scared and depressed.

I returned him to school and on my way back I heard the end of a Paul Harvey broadcast about a doctor treating asthma and allergies with water! My initial reaction was skeptical. As I started my son on medications I kept remembering that broadcast. Within 2 days of beginning medications he felt worse. His mouth and throat burned, the medicine made him irritable, drowsy and sun-sensitive. At this point I decided to investigate this broadcast further. I called the main office of Paul Harvey News and a very helpful woman looked up the broadcast and gave me the phone number to contact Global Health Solutions. I contacted them immediately and they were also very helpful. I ordered Dr. F. Batmanghelidj's book *Your Body's Many Cries for Water*. I was also given a phone number to call Dr. Batmanghelidj if desired. The book arrived a few days later; I started my son on Dr. B.'s recommended rehydration program with a little added salt and after less than a week, his symptoms have almost completely stopped and he is feeling great and taking NO medications!!

The information and help given us by Dr. Batmanghelidj saved our family much emotional and financial distress that could have gone on for years. Please pass this information to others. My son was ill and that distressed us, but many children actually DIE from this condition every year!!

In a Paul Harvey editorial of January 24, 1994, in the *Connecticut Post* he wrote: "I don't know if Dr. Fereydoon Batmanghelidj's idea is worth anything or not," also "maybe this doctor is just another opportunist selling books, but on the chance that he has something, let's listen . . ." I can tell you most assuredly that his "idea" is WORTH MUCH! It makes a great deal of sense and is utterly simple and totally effective. I can also attest that he is absolutely not an opportunist selling books. I admit I was skeptical initially. Since my receipt of his book I wrote him a note to thank him and shortly thereafter received a personal phone call from him offering help and assistance at any time. He then followed up a few days later to check my son's progress and again offer help. AND HIS PRESCRIPTION WAS WORKING!!

Dr. Batmanghelidj has committed himself to get this information to the public in whatever way he can. The medical profession will not listen; he has tried that. It is a terrible crime that so many are suffering when the solution is so simple and readily obtainable. Dr. Batmanghelidj's research and commitment is truly a gift and applies to us all!!!!

Please help pass on this information to anyone you can! I am committed to doing just that.
Sincerely, C. W. B.

◊   ◊   ◊

Asthma:

Dear Dr. Batmanghelidj,

I would like to give you my story on how your therapy of drinking water has helped my health. You are free to use this letter as you see fit.

I suffered from a severe case of asthma and allergies my whole life. As a child, I was treated with allergy shots which provided no relief. I found asthma inhalers a constant companion. In fact, I could not be anywhere without an inhaler or risk a severe asthma attack. During this same time I also had a terrible case of allergic rhinitis.

I was miserable during the spring, summer and fall seasons. When I entered medical school, I received some relief of my symptoms from steroid inhalers, both for my lungs and my nasal passages. By using these inhalers throughout the day, I was much more comfortable. But I still found it impossible to be without a daily inhaler for my asthma.

Nowhere in my medical training was it stressed to me the importance of drinking water to control these diseases (or any other conditions). I was thoroughly trained on pharmacology and the "wonders" of drug therapies. Shortly after I finished my residency, I read a review of your book, *Your Body's Many Cries for Water*. Though I was skeptical your ideas could help me overcome my illness, I decided to get this book.

When I read the book, the simplicity of your hypothesis made complete sense to me. When I realized the coffee and soda that I was drinking were actually leaving me in a dehydrated state, I could begin to understand why I was suffering from asthma and allergies. I immediately began drinking more water and stopped drinking non-water sources.

Within a short time, I began to feel better. My asthma symptoms markedly improved and my allergy symptoms diminished. Though I still had to use my inhalers, I was able to significantly decrease the dosage of medication. I was very pleased with the results, and began recommending this therapy to my patients.

Approximately two years later, I was preparing to give a speech on acupuncture. I decided to tell the audience about the benefits of water, so I read your book again. This time, I noticed the section on the importance of salt. I had almost totally omitted salt from my diet. When I added a pinch of sea salt to my regimen, ALL OF MY SYMPTOMS OF ASTHMA AND ALLERGIES RESOLVED WITHIN TWO DAYS! For the first time in my life, I am now free of all medications and I feel wonderful. Your work has changed my practice and made me a better physician.

Thank you.
Sincerely, David Brownstein, M.D.

**Migraines; Constipation; Nosebleeds;
Allergies: Asthma:**

I live in Oregon's Willamette Valley. According to my allergist, this is one of the worst places in the nation for allergy sufferers. For years I had taken antihistamines year-round for multiple environmental allergies, along with steroid nose sprays and inhalers for asthma. I took allergy shots for a period of five years. After all that, I still had allergy symptoms in the spring, summer and fall when not taking antihistamines daily. Last year, my 2 1/2-year old daughter was diagnosed with allergies and asthma and placed on antihistamines and inhalers as well.

Then, along came the book *Your Body's Many Cries for Water.* When my wife introduced me to your book in August 1998, I was very skeptical. I have a master's degree in clinical social work and have been trained that medications are an integral part of managing most chronic illnesses. However, your presentation on the importance of water and the dehydrating effects of medications made sense. For me, constipation, bloody nose and migraines were frequent side effects of the dehydration intensified by allergy and asthma medications.

After reading your book, my daughter and I stopped taking medications. My daughter and I began drinking the suggested amounts of water, supplementing it with sea salt. Having read elsewhere about the effects of dairy on allergies and asthma, we also eliminated dairy products from our diet. My daughter's asthma and allergy symptoms immediately went away. My symptoms were greatly reduced, and with careful attention to my water and salt intake, and by eliminating dairy from my diet, I have rarely experienced allergy and asthma symptoms and no longer suffer the uncomfortable side effects of medications.

Thank you for bringing to light this commonsense remedy.
Sincerely, J. B.

Allergies; Hypertension:

I would like to give you a quick update to the success of the hydration program I have been following for the last several years. I am almost totally free from the severe allergic reactions I suffered from all my life. When I do have a reaction it is mild and short, and I enjoy the side benefit that I am almost never sick with the flu or colds. The most beneficial effect of this program has been to keep my hypertension condition under acceptable parameters. Your advice several years ago has significantly improved the quality and duration of my life. I am a grateful and devoted student of your principles of hydration. I would like to thank you for your continued devotion to the study of the healing properties of proper hydration.
Sincerely, M. A. P.

Cholesterol; Allergies:

I had been suffering from an allergy-related affliction for more than a year when I discovered your new paradigm in modern medicine, specifically the consumption of two quarts of water a day as the basis for better health.

I've been practicing your program for almost six months. My water intake is now 8–10 glasses a day. I've added salt back into my diet (which you point out is especially important for allergy/asthma sufferers), and changed my exercise regimen by adding daily walks. I also deleted caffeinated coffee from my diet.

The results are very encouraging. I'm experiencing increased strength and vigor and was amazed and grateful when I recently learned that my blood cholesterol has decreased from 229 to 159. I was also somewhat surprised that even with the re-introduction of salt into my diet six months ago, my blood pressure is 108/70.

Thank you for all of the efforts you've made to bring these important ideas to the attention of public health professionals and society-at-large.
Sincerely, W. M.

Allergies; Excess Mucus:

I discovered your wonderful book on "water as medicine" while taking a three-month course on commodities trading from the Ken Roberts Company. One of his many other business interests is Four Star Books (mostly dealing with books on spiritual insight). Their one-page advertisement enticed me to order *Your Body's Many Cries for Water.*

I wrote to Ken personally and told him that your book alone was worth the price of his course. Allow me to explain:

I've been suffering from an allergy-related affliction for almost a year and a half. Since about age eight I have had seasonal allergic rhinitis, due (I thought) to the high pollen counts here in northern California's Santa Clara Valley (better known these days as "Silicon Valley"). A year ago February, I picked up a virus that was making the rounds here in the valley. Symptoms included a cough with excess mucus that created a kind of "lump in the throat." Since I'm usually in excellent health (I've used my Kaiser Health Plan facility less than half a dozen times in 15 years—for check-ups, vasectomy, and allergy-related problems) I waited until April to see a doctor. I hoped these symptoms would clear up on their own.

An RN told me this virus was widespread, contagious and she had suffered from it herself, on and off, at least three times. She prescribed three different medications (two pills and a nasal inhaler). I tried out the prescriptions, but found that the side effects produced additional problems and the relief seemed to be only partial. I stopped taking the medications on my own after about three weeks. My initial reaction was that "they're only treating the symptoms! I want a cure that will alleviate the cause of this problem."

I began to change my diet to include more fruits and vegetables and non-mucus-forming foods. I cut way down on meat and dairy products and this helped, but only somewhat.

By February 1997 the problem of excess mucus in my lungs had not improved and so, frustrated, I returned to Kaiser and worked with an

MD who is a specialist in internal medicine. She prescribed an oral inhaler. This helped me overcome some of the early symptoms of spring allergies, but nothing helped alleviate the symptom of excess mucus in my lungs. My lungs had become really sore from over a year of coping with my seriously dehydrated condition. In addition, the discomforts of excess mucus worked to curb my appetite and I lost 10–15 pounds during this period as my weight fell to 135 lbs on a 5' 10" slender frame. Clearly my health was in serious jeopardy.

It's now July 9, 1997. I read your book three weeks ago and began to take many of the steps that you recommend. I stopped drinking coffee immediately. I now drink only one cup of decaf coffee in the morning. I've cut my consumption of wine in half and I've increased the salt in my diet. Interesting enough, I've used almost no salt for years, believing the current trend in medical thinking that salt causes high blood pressure and is harmful to the body. Most importantly, I'm drinking 8–10 glasses of water a day as you suggest. I'm walking twice a day as well.

What a difference!! I still have excess mucus. However, in three short weeks it's about half of what I've experienced in the past year and a half. My worst day now is better that my best day before. My appetite has improved, my energy level is increasing and I find myself more centered and focused in the "here and now." I know as I continue this "life-style change" and re-hydrate my body I'll improve even more over time. I tell myself that I can't expect to heal the problems of a lifetime in a few short weeks. I'm now 49 years old. I've probably been dehydrated since my youth. My affliction was no doubt my body's attempt to tell me I was severely dehydrated.

Almost as important as symptom relief are the renewed feelings of underlying health that accompany this program. The mental and emotional frustrations of dealing with a medical establishment bent on treating symptoms without understanding the root causes of disease are almost as debilitating as the disease itself.

I apologize for dwelling on myself in this letter, but I thought you would appreciate a detailed account of my experience. The real purpose of my contacting you is to thank you for your continued efforts at educating about water as medicine and your extreme dedication and perseverance to your work. Your attempts to change the medical "status quo" in the face of adversity are exemplary. I know that your work has changed my life, as well as countless others, for the better.

Thank you again for your valuable contributions to the individual and collective health of this world.
Sincerely, W. M.

◊   ◊   ◊

Depression; Allergies:

For as long as I can remember, I have suffered from allergic rhinitis, and have been sporadically treated with anti-histamine drugs for many years. I have also suffered from depression for the last four years, which lifted slightly from time to time, but always returned. A friend mentioned the story of Dr. Batman's discovery of the amazing potential of water to 'treat' many different illnesses. Having noted in the past that when I increased my water intake and decreased caffeine I felt much better, I decided to investigate further.

Five days into my healthy new life, and I feel so different. The allergic rhinitis would appear to have completely vanished, and the depression seems so much improved, that I'm tempted to say that that, too, has vanished. How utterly incredible!!!!!

Dr. Batman—thank you, so much, for your research and for your hard work in bringing this to the attention of the public. It is a wonderful, life-changing "treatment"—at absolutely no cost!!
Thank you again.
Sincerely, J. J.,
Dorset, England

Bronchitis; Breathing Difficulty:

Again, I wish to thank you for helping me to better appreciate the importance of water to my health. In May of this year, I acquired a sinus infection followed by bronchitis in June. Both were treated medically and apparently successfully. The following month while vacationing in the high country of New Mexico, I developed difficulty in breathing to the point that I cut my vacation short to consult with my doctor.

The problem seemed to be shortness of breath or insufficient intake of air. My doctor immediately referred me to the hospital for a series of tests in view of my breathing problem and the previous sinus and bronchitis that I had experienced. In the hospital my lungs were X-rayed, oxygen content in my blood tested, EKG, stress tested, heart monitored for twenty-four hours, and my lungs were scanned. Tests revealed nothing. On the third day, I was released and was prescribed Xanax to be taken whenever a "breathing incident" occurred. My breathing difficulty remained unchanged.

A friend with whom my husband had discussed my hospital visit and problem visited us and shared the issue *The Last Chance Health Report* health newsletter, volume 3, #5, in which Sam Biser reported his interview with you, in the article, "The True Unknown Cause and Cure of Asthma."

As soon as I finished reading the article I started the water treatment and have been on it since early August. Let me emphasize that I had become very inactive and spoke as little as possible since my breathing became difficult. Within one week of drinking at least eight glasses of water daily my breathing became easier and less labored. I regained my normal energy. For over three weeks of this date I have been walking three miles in the morning and three miles in the evenings. I have not taken the Xanax as I detest tranquilizers, nor have I been on any other medication. I have since secured a copy of your book *Your Body's Many Cries for Water,* read it, and shared it with friends and relatives.

It is my prayer that other people with breathing problems read about you and try the water treatment that has helped me so much.
With best wishes!
Sincerely, M. A.

Asthma:

I appreciate your invite to call you. I feel this letter will better sum up what I have to say than my jabbering over the phone.

I've got big news for you. After 30 years of suffering with asthma, I think I have been cured . . . I'm not kidding you . . . . CURED!

While browsing the Internet, I came upon a site called watercure.com and watercure2.com.

They reasoned that asthma could be cured by water and salt intake. I was skeptical, but also at the end of my rope, having suffered this debilitating disease for most of my life. I was wheezing so bad that it was either give this a try or go into Emergency . . . . again . . . .

Within 2 days my symptoms disappeared. I've been asthma free for 8 days now. I haven't needed to use my inhaler once during that time, and IT IS NOTHING SHORT OF A MIRACLE what I've experienced.

I believe your products are well intentioned. . . . and I'm sure they help. . . but as a long-time suffering asthmatic I IMPLORE you: if you really care about the suffering of your clients you will direct them to the aforementioned websites and encourage them to try this water and salt therapy. It's free and it WORKS.

As I've stated, I've experienced a miracle. NEVER before have I achieved such impressive results; prednisone, inhalers, nebulizers—you name it— have never given me as much relief as drinking water and taking salt.

Just so you know, I'm not your everyday run-of-the-mill asthmatic. I've probably been in the emergency room at least 100 times throughout my life, and admitted probably 30 times. I've tried it all. This is the first "natural" therapy that I've tried that actually worked. I feel as though I've been given a new lease on life. I'm hoping you share my discovery with your patients.

I gain nothing by this. The water cure is free. All they ask is that you tell anyone and everyone who will listen about the miracle of water and salt

therapy. I'm doing my share in the hopes that maybe there will be one less asthmatic in the world.
Hopefully you will keep in touch.
Best wishes, Mike

        💧   💧   💧

Asthma; Breathing Difficulty:

I am so happy that I came across your book, *Your Body's Many Cries for Water*. I work at a public library and just happened to pick up a recent copy of *Publisher's Weekly* Magazine, and saw an ad for your book. It captured my attention immediately, although I didn't really know why at the time. I am 60 years old, and have been reasonably healthy all my life, but the past few years, I have been plagued with symptoms of asthma—difficulty breathing, bouts with coughing, and of course, many nights of interrupted sleep, if not completely sleepless. I tried cough-medicines, throat lozenges, and nasal sprays, dietary changes, all to no avail.

Last winter (Feb 2000) I was diagnosed with a mild case of pneumonia, and was in considerable pain and discomfort with that. A course of strong antibiotics eventually cleared it up, but the asthmatic symptoms never really went away. When I got a copy of your book a few weeks ago I was fascinated immediately by what you have to say about the body's dehydration and it certainly made sense to me. I hadn't been drinking water in years, just coffee, juices, and tea, thinking that that had to be enough liquid. Clearly it wasn't, as I continued to read and learn about asthma onset.

I am in my fourth week of water-therapy, as I call it, and I have to say I am in much better shape. The coughing and excess mucus is subsiding, I'm sleeping for an uninterrupted eight hours a night, and overall I just feel MUCH better! I took note of the need for increased salt intake as part of the program. I am SO grateful to you for this simple solution to some pretty severe problems for a lot of people. Thank you so much for your research and work on this, and for the courage and vision to continue it under clearly unfriendly, even hostile, circumstances.

You can be sure I am spreading the word in whatever way I can, but mostly, just following your guidelines is what is really going to change a lot of people's lives.
Sincere thanks! S. C.

P.S. I would be happy to have this testimonial posted on your website, or included in any printed material you wish to publish.

♦   ♦   ♦

**Bronchiectasis; Cough;
Rash; Shortness of Breath:**

I am so grateful for your book. I heard about *Your Body's Many Cries for Water* through the Ken Roberts Company. I am writing to you concerning my husband Gene, 58, who have bronchiectasis. Ever since his many sinus surgeries, starting back in 1984, he has had trouble with his respiratory functions. This past June he became really sick. He couldn't breathe, was fatigued, and had a constant cough. X-rays were taken and misread. Referrals to specialists take time and are not always easy to get in this land of HMOs. Now in September, Gene finally saw a specialist who said he had been walking around with pneumonia since June. He also broke out in a rash all over his body. I have never seen anything like it—he was covered!! Gene has been living on antibiotics for years and now they are not working anymore. The specialist admitted him to the hospital for intravenous administration of antibiotics.

This is where you come in, Dr. B. I was reading your book at the time Gene went to the hospital, and I started him on the water program while he was in hospital. I am telling you I saw the results within 24 hours!! The most noticeable was the cough. Suddenly he wasn't constantly coughing anymore, just once in a while and then it didn't sound so deep in his chest. It was all up-hill from there!! I'm sure the antibiotics were helping too, but I still think it was the water that brought him around so quickly. He is continuing your program, incorporating the salt as well into his diet.

I mentioned this to the doctor who agreed about the importance of water, but that was the end of it. It's like you said: only if one is on the verge of collapsing from dehydration does one do anything about it. The doctors never considered hydrating Gene, but many thanks to you, I did!! My hope and intent is to one day have Gene off all medication. Thank you again,
Sincerely, M. M.

Bursitis; Allergies; Heartburn:

Please accept the following statement as a testimonial to the water cure:

I started the Water Cure to relieve nagging lower back pain. Not only did it cure that, it cured bursitis I had in my shoulder, eliminated my need to take antacids for my stomach and antihistamines I was taking for chronic allergies, and if that was not enough, I no longer have dandruff; and, it lowered my cholesterol and blood pressure, but someone might think I am stretching the truth. I'm not!
Thank you.
Sincerely, T. J.

Cholesterol:

The only purpose of this letter is to express to you my deepest feelings of gratitude for having conveyed to your readers the healing virtues and gist of the simplest of all elements: water. It is really *elixir vitae!* I don't exaggerate in saying that you are a benefactor of humanity. May millions and millions apply your incredible discovery.

I am 75 years old, my health has wonderfully improved, the cholesterol level is again normal, since I've strictly followed your advice—the more willingly since we have in our village one of the best waters in Europe:

Evian water directly from the source. . . .
Again my wholehearted thanks for favors received through you. God
bless you.
Prof. D. Rene Lejeune
France

P.S. I spread the good news through my writings.

♦   ♦   ♦

Cholesterol:

This is to say how grateful I am to you for making me a much less worried
man. I have suffered from a high cholesterol level since 1982. It was 278
when it was first discovered. I was then in Germany and I was put on such a
strict diet that I lost 16 pounds in less than two months and the cholesterol
level went down to only 220. I refused to accept to lower it further through
medication especially since in Egypt the doctors still believe that this level is
not really dangerous by the prevailing standards in our country.

Since I entertain and attend business lunches more than what would be
expected even from a diplomat, because of the additional burden of dealing
with the media, my cholesterol was always going up to around 260 and back
to 220, by putting myself on very strict diet from time to time. However, it
must be noted that it was only outside my home that the diet came crashing
down; otherwise, I was strict with myself. In fact, even when I ate outside, I
was careful to choose dishes, wherever available, which were not particularly rich in fat.

Last year I was shocked to discover that my blood cholesterol level had shot
up to 279. I was lucky to have met you then. When you "prescribed" ample
water (two full glasses) be taken before meals instead of medication that I
was just about to submit myself to then, I was very skeptical. All the more so
since you did not overemphasize dieting. In two months and with very little
observance of all the old "rules" which were making my life miserable my
cholesterol went down to 203 for the first time in more than nine years! My
weight too was surprisingly also down by about eight pounds and has since
been under control.

Enjoying eating moderately of course, as I had not been doing for a long time and free from a worry that was always at the back of my mind, I believe I owe you a big THANK YOU!
Sincerely yours,
Minister M. W.
Director, Press and Information Bureau

◆ ◆ ◆

Migraine; Neck and Shoulder Pain; Abdominal Pain:

I am a 37-year-old female who has never been thirsty. At 22, I was diagnosed with high cholesterol (256) with no other "symptoms." I used to joke with all of my friends that I must have been from a "desert people" in a previous life because I never felt like drinking water. The joking stopped a few weeks ago when I found myself almost too weak to move. My hips, shoulders, lower back and neck were sore, my head was pounding and my tongue was swollen! As I lay there wondering, "why me?" I realized I had not had any plain water in over three days! In that moment I realized I had the power to choose life (water) or to continue to die a slow and painful death.

The first glass made me feel like a wilted flower coming back to life. After that first glass, I started to do research into my lack of thirst, water deprivation and, finally, chronic dehydration. I was shocked that something so simple could explain away all my various health problems over the years. I've complained at one time or another to various healthcare professionals of: migraine headaches, high cholesterol, pain in my left knee, stomach pain/ulcers, etc. I ordered and read *Your Body's Many Cries for Water*. Thank you for taking this well-meaning and necessary stand! I continue to struggle every day to drink my required water. It is still so foreign to me! In any event, after the first few days of full water intake, I felt almost giddy and was "floating." My body is adapting to my increased water intake slowly and though some days I don't drink all my required water, I am now fully cognizant of my water needs and intake. I feel better and seem to have more energy, although I know I still have a full two months until I'm fully rehydrated.

Now, I am working on a freelance article about chronic dehydration for a women's health and fitness magazine. I would like some information on calculating a body's true daily water needs. I am using the basic 1/2 body weight in ounces of water per day calculation but am concerned that this amount doesn't take into consideration the additional needs a woman's body may have (a) at various times in her cycle, (b) after strenuous exercise, and (c) during pregnancy/nursing.

Also, as a side issue (and perhaps a follow-up piece for a parenting magazine), what is the best way to calculate true water needs for a child or infant? I truly believe that if we can teach our children to drink the proper amount of water, they can avoid the pain and dis-ease of past generations.

Any assistance you can give will be greatly appreciated. Respectfully, R. B. L.

Note: A child needs more water than a grown person. The reason is obvious: Every new cell in the body of a developing child needs to be filled with 75 percent of its volume with water. Filling each cell in the body of a growing child is what "growth" is about. A pregnant mother needs to drink more good-quality water than other people to supply the fetus in her uterus. Good-quality water does not mean manufactured beverages and alcohol that further dehydrate the body. The dehydration of the mother could be stressful to the fetus and establish the "chemistry of anxiety" in the child even after birth. This is why children of alcoholics are prone to serious health problems later in life.

From birth to full growth, the body of a child still needs more water than grown people. As you noticed in the letters on asthma, water is essential to prevent diseases of dehydration, which include the autoimmune diseases such as insulin-dependent diabetes, fibrocystic diseases, lupus, and more. Infants need water, too. Whereas the mother's milk is dilute, formula milk may not have enough water and may produce an array of problems such as unexplained earaches and respiratory problems that might have to be viewed as infantile asthma, which I consider to be the cause of SIDS (sudden infant death syndrome, sometimes known as crib death or cot death). Children have a very acute sensation of thirst. The main problem is their choice of "fluids" in place of the simple water their bodies are designed to process.

Water should be introduced into the diet of infants to prevent them from getting dehydrated, which *strongly, chemically, physiologically, directly, and indirectly suppresses their immune system at its bone marrow level of functions*. It does not take much water to prevent dehydration in infants. A few ounces daily, added to their formula milk composition throughout the day, might be enough. Mothers should cultivate children's taste for simple water. This would be the greatest act of love for their offspring. The water you add to the formula milk will generate energy for growth—yes, water is the primary source of energy for all chemical functions of the body; it generates hydro-electricity at all the cell membranes in the body—and the solid components of the milk would then be used for construction of new tissues.

At a conference where I talked and explained the relationship of low water consumption to cholesterol deposits in the heart arteries, an English physician told me about the outcome of autopsies in infants who died in car accidents. The ones on mother's milk had clear coronary arteries. The infants on formula showed fairly serious blockage in some of the arteries of their heart. This alone indicates that infants should be given more water than is customary now.

Hypertension; Diabetes:

Thank you for your comment. My patients are improving a lot with water and salt. I'm doing that with the patients with high blood pressure, excellent results now but I was a little scared with the first one. Now, I'm more confident and am using this with diabetic people, type 2 and type 1.

Thank you again.
Marco Vinicio Velasquez Monge

Diabetes; Weight Loss;
Sleep; Anxiety:

I have only you to thank for how terrific I feel. Several months ago, I read an article on your research on water. Not being sick at the time, I didn't follow your advice. On June 1, after telling my father I thought I was dehydrated, he tested my blood sugar—it was 465. I immediately went to the doctor at which time she grimly stated the pills might not work. I recalled your article and set out to cure myself with water. How much water I thought?? I didn't know so I chose a gallon a day. I am ecstatic to say 2 1/2 weeks later I was pill free! I have spread the word to anyone who is willing to listen. My father, an insulin-dependent diabetic, has been drinking water for a month and says he feels great too. My readings are usually under 125 and have not gone past 139; I have lost weight, sleep better, have less anxiety and just feel great.

My only wish is to extend my gratitude for your perseverance in educating people on the benefits of water, and the new approach to medicine. God Bless, L. L.

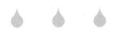

Diabetes; Weight Loss:

I cannot get hold of the Dr. who publishes the water cure, but maybe you can tell him—Thank you so very, very much!

I developed diabetes type-2. My glucose reading at the time was 560 with 100+/- being the norm. My doctor almost killed me by over-medicating me with injectable insulin. A new doctor put me on Glucophage twice per day. Then I found the "Water Cure" from a group in England. I believed Dr. B. said that it would take two months—it took three. My glucose readings are in the normal range, 87–115 fasting. I just cannot believe I am free of the diabetes.

I still have problems with occluded arteries, which preceded the diabetes, but I am working on that. I am aghast at how many suffer and die from diabetes and it can be cured. I drink at least 10 glasses of water a day. I am so tickled that I am going to live and not suffer from the disease or heart attack or brain attack.

This simple cure saved my life—how profoundly grateful I am. My wife drinks water now too. She was obese but has steadily been losing weight.

Thank you for what you are doing.
May God bless you, Sean

**Weight Loss; Diabetes;
Asthma; Back Pain:**

Our E.A.P. specialist has been on the water program for about seven weeks. He weighed in at 295; he's presently lost 40 pounds; he's lost all traces of diabetes; his asthma has been noticeably relieved, and his skin has improved.

He now plays golf without back pain, and incidentally, this is very important to him. He's the biggest enthusiast we have and as you know, as an E.A.P. specialist, he's in the field contacting the people covered by our Insurance Trust daily, in that his specialty is drug addiction and alcoholism. He's taken many of our tapes, quite a few of our books and is promoting the program personally.

I've been on the program for quite a while and I feel that my indigestion has improved, my taste far more precise and overall I feel it's working. The same situation holds true for P.G., our insurance manager, a young guy in his thirties, and to my knowledge, he is very, very pleased with the results of the water cure so far. Will keep you posted. Once again, thank you for all your efforts and dedication.
Sincerely, A. S.

Diabetes:

Six months after reading the material on the water cure given to me by Bob Butts, I was diagnosed with diabetes. In talking to Bob, he encouraged me to try this method to cure my problem. Of course like many others, I was skeptical of how water could do very much to eliminate this disease. My blood glucose level was about 240 and the other problems of frequent urination, constant hunger and constant thirst. I did as your information advised and visited my doctor. He recommended pills, but I convinced him that we should try your regimen for a few months before trying medication.

After about ten weeks and a loss of forty pounds, my blood sugar levels are now between 110 and 125. I do watch them at least once or twice a day. I still have not taken any medication, but do watch the food intake closely.

Please have anyone call who would like to discuss my results.
Very truly yours,
Lubeco Inc. J. B. P. 3rd.

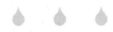

Diabetes:

I am providing you herewith a detailed and complete history of morning fasting blood sugar readings for my 40-year-old disabled daughter Susan, who earlier this year was diagnosed with maturity-onset diabetes, and started on your recommended water and sea salt regime starting on 5/14/98. As the attached chart shows, we were first alerted about her blood sugar problem on 5/5/98, when "routine" blood tests showed a random reading of 298 mg/dl. Prompt follow-up morning fasting tests yielded readings of 189 mg/dl on 5/7/98 and a double-checking 159 mg/dl (also fasting) on 5/20/98. However, after the first fasting reading, she got started promptly on the water and salt—before the second fasting test. Her AIC reading of 9.4 (also 5/7/98) left little doubt in the doctor's mind about the certainty of the diagnosis of diabetes.

In the first three months with water and salt, her morning fasting blood sugar averaged approximately 133 mg/dl, showing a good regulation for a diabetic, and at the end of these first three months her AIC improved to 7.1, measured on 9/3/98. She has had no AIC test since 9/3/98 but her fasting blood sugar readings have continued to improve, averaging approximately 114 mg/dl from 9/3/98 to the present time, showing strong evidence that the next AIC will no doubt show significant additional improvement. The morning fasting blood sugar readings were plotted individually on the chart, but a 20-day moving average of these readings was also plotted for clarity of interpretation.

It is significant that in achieving these improved fasting blood sugar readings, Susan received no insulin nor other medications, and that rather than being on a strict diet, she followed the same "normal" perhaps quite typical eating habits of the rest of the household, with one exception. She and also my wife and I tended to eat out even less often, although we never did eat out any more often than once every 4 to 6 weeks or so even before Susan's diabetes evidenced itself. Since then it has been even less frequent.

A week ago yesterday I attended a diabetes support group meeting at which the guest speaker was a recently retired endocrinologist who headed the diabetic department at our HMO for several years. The subject of his talk was nerve degeneration in diabetics, how to minimize it, etc. After the meeting I showed him Susan's graphic record of blood sugar readings. He got all excited and said this was phenomenal. In reply to his asking, I told him Susan was following the program in your book, *Your Body's Many Cries for Water.* When he asked how he could get the book, I produced my personal copy and he promptly bought it from me. Hopefully, this detailed record of Susan's case will be a helpful addition in your research efforts. Susan has happily consented to your using this data in your researches, and also as appropriate, in your future writings. Thanks much for your help.
Sincerely, T. P.

Hypertension:

You wrote a small article on "Water" in the book *Amazing Medicines* by University Medical Research Publication, which has helped me, lower my blood count and blood pressure considerably.

Thank you very much for all your good work.
Sincerely, B. M.

Hypertension; Cholesterol:

I am writing to give you a report on how drinking more water each day has improved my health. I started drinking eight to ten glasses of water last July 1994 after reading your paper on *Your Body's Many Cries for Water.* After being on this extra water for six months, I have reduced my blood pressure from 140 over 80 to 110 over 70. Also, my cholesterol level has gone from 201 to 171. I have noticed that my weight has stabilized. I always put on about four to five pounds during the fall. That has not happened. The only change in my diet has been the water intake.

Another interesting report, I now take a glass of water each night to my nightstand. Almost every night, in the early hours, my body cries for water. I become very dry and thirsty.

I look forward to receiving your autographed book. I think it will be easier to convince people that water intake will make a difference for them.
Sincerely, B. P.

Hypertension:

Since my 24 May 1994 letter and your consequent telephone call, a physical change of address has absorbed my time.

Albeit, much more important than these facts, I am in a position to verify how tap water effectively lowers hypertension. Starting in early April 1994, leaving years of diuretics and calcium-blockers behind, in accordance with your recommendation, for approximately 3 months I drank a minimum of eight 8-ounce glasses of tap water, occasionally more. The blood pressure, heretofore contained by drugs, gradually dropped from an average around 150–160 systolic/over 95–98 diastolic to an amazing, *DRUG FREE* 130–135 systolic/over 75–80 diastolic fluctuating averages.

My wife makes these measurements at home; each time taking two or three readings. The record shows several lows of 120 systolic over 75 diastolic and a rare high of 140 systolic over 90 diastolic. However, the average range, as stated above uniformly dominates.

In addition to vitamins and minerals, this drug-free approach, based essentially on tap water and a pinch of salt, has relaxed my system and justifies the confidence that you hold the handles of a truly revolutionary and marvelous medical concept.

Since you are about to publish a book with applicable testimonies of the hydration system, my personal experience is gratefully offered as a way of saying thank you.
Respectfully yours, W. F. B.
Lt. Col. AUS RET

◆ ◆ ◆

Hypertension:

I discovered the importance of water and salt to the human body in June of 1997 when I failed a medical for renewing my commercial flying license. My pressure at rest was 230/110. I was grounded and told to see my personal physician. He told me I needed blood pressure medication, but I decided I was not going on any medication yet.

I left upset, in denial. My blood pressure had always been 120/80. I got second opinion weeks later after trying garlic, herbs, vitamins, exercise, medication and found it still a solid 180/100. He told me if I didn't go on medication, my heart would enlarge and I would have a heart attack or stroke down the road.

I went home depressed. I didn't want to accept old age at 54. I was telling a friend about my situation when a retired chiropractor told me about your book (*Your Body's Many Cries for Water*). He loaned me his book and told me to stop all caffeine for a week, drink ten glasses of water and add 1/2 tsp. of salt to my diet.

I looked at him like he was crazy. I had been on a salt-free diet for years. Thank God for your book Dr. Batmanghelidj and Dr. Lee Hobson for his time and generosity.

My blood pressure is now 117/75. I'm taking no medication at all and I have unlimited energy at 56 years old. No more headache or lower back pain; sinuses are clear and no constipation.
Thankfully, Jim Bolen

Note: I leave Jim's name at the bottom of his letter in order to acknowledge him for his unceasing efforts during the past number of years to share the story of water with people he comes across. He has used truck driving across America, from north to south and west to east on major highways, making contact at truck stops, at churches, at locations he delivers his goods, and through his radio communications with his fellow drivers to share his knowledge of water with whomever listens to him. He has developed such a command of the subject that he even confounds me whenever we meet.

By now, he must have reached tens of thousands of people. He has allocated a major portion of his income to buying books, videos, and audiotapes to give out to churches and people who need more information. He gives them the educational materials as loans, but seldom gets them back. He has assigned himself the responsibility of becoming a missionary to help innocent and uninsured people achieve a naturally better health and escape the ever-stretched claws of the sick-care system. I have come across quite a number of people who have been saved by Jim. He is well known among his peers in the trucking profession. May God bless him for his noble undertaking.

Neck Pain; Blood Pressure:

Collegial greetings and I again wish to thank you for the work you are doing trying to get out the word on chronic dehydration. I have personally received great benefit from this information during the past five weeks. I am spreading the word in my retirement community and have had several converts. With my order of two books I enclosed a letter addressed to you personally, but I don't know whether you received it. I will include a copy with this.

Since I began trying to drink eighty ounces (wt. is 160#) water per day these are the changes I noted.

Within the first 48 hours my need for acetaminophen had decreased from an average of 2 grams daily to zero. About the third day I noticed I was having lightheaded feelings and checked my BP out at 92/45, whereupon I reduced my Monopril from 15 mgm/day to 10 mgm/day and my BP has stabilized at 110/55. I lost some weight (edema) so reduced my diuretic Maxzide from 75/37.5 down to 37.5/25 and continue to do okay. I'm working with my doctor to see if we can reduce my meds any further. Prior to this my BP has run 120/70 most of my life.

I am currently on Lanoxin 0.125-mgm; Maxzide 37.5/25; Monopril 10-mgm; atenolol 50-mgm; and Pravachol 20-mgm and ASA 80-mgm daily. My hope is that I will be able to reduce some of those and perhaps even discontinue them in time.

They tell me that I have left ventricular insufficiency due to a markedly enlarged heart resulting from the loss of heart muscle after two major MI's in 1980 and 1990. Had six-vessel by-pass in 1990. My edema fluctuates between 1 and 2 plus in spite of spending several hours daily with my feet elevated, and up to 3–4 when I am on my feet more. I experience one-flight dyspnea and can walk one half mile with some difficulty—but no angina.

Also I wanted to report that I have found the pain in my neck to be a very good indicator of dehydration. When I don't get enough water one day I begin the very next morning to have a return of pain and within an hour or two of drinking a few glasses of water the pain goes away. I have taken no pain Rx for the past month since I started on the water routine.

Keep up the good work and may God bless you in your crusade,
Donald P. Jackson, M.D.

💧   💧   💧

Hypertension; Allergies; Asthma:

Just wanted to write you a quick note to thank you for your book *Your Body's Many Cries for Water*. After reading this book, I remarked to my wife "this guy is a genius"! Who could have guessed that all these seemingly unrelated medical problems could all be tied to dehydration?

For years, my blood pressure was borderline high and I was drinking way too much coffee and not enough water. Within days of stopping coffee, my blood pressure improved dramatically. Starting to drink more water has further normalized it. I have gone from readings of 134/93 to as low as 118/78 in as little as a month.

In addition, I think dehydration was causing a wide range of other problems for me such as allergies and asthma. I really look forward to see how much I can improve on your "regimen."

One quick question, if you would be so kind. I have recently become quite interested in the heart-protecting and other qualities of garlic and/or garlic supplements. Now, I suspect the one problem with them is that they may have a diuretic property. Is it OK to use garlic in this fashion if I am consuming no other substance like coffee, tea, sodas etc. (drinking plenty of water)?

Once again, thank you so much for your book. You told me what years of visiting doctors failed to. I earnestly believe you may have saved me from a lifetime of unnecessarily poor health!
Regards, D. B.

Hypertension; Weight Loss:

This letter is a testimony to the merits of water as an essential part of the daily dietary requirements for good health. I have been following your recommendations for nearly five years, and have found myself taking for granted the positive effects of water intake.

When I first started on the program I was overweight, with high blood pressure and suffering from asthma and allergies, which I have had since a small child. I had been receiving treatment for these conditions. Today, I have my weight and blood pressure under control (weight loss of approximately 30 pounds and a 10 point drop in blood pressure). The program reduced the frequency of asthma and allergy-related problems, to the point of practical nonexistence. Additionally, there were other benefits. I experienced fewer colds, and flu, generally with less severity.

I introduced this program to my wife, who had been on blood pressure medication for the past four years, and through increased water intake she has recently been able to eliminate her medication.

Thanks again for your program, M. P.

Polycythemia; Hypertension:

Several months ago I finished reading your fascinating book *Your Body's Many Cries for Water.* I truly have to say that I couldn't put it down until I finished reading it. Several of my friends and family members have also read it. My brother, who has some medical background, has also read it, and he found it very interesting.

I have a medical condition called Polycythemia Vera. My body produces too many red blood cells. I am on medication called hydroxyurea. Also from time to time they have to do a phlebotomy on me. I was diagnosed with this illness about nine years ago when I was 33 years old, but my doctor said that probably I had the illness several years before that. It is a rare illness usually occurring in much older people. People of my age usually do not have this illness. Nobody knows what causes this illness. I was told perhaps stress has something to do with it. Also, I used to be a security guard for several years and I worked in factories and industrial sites and perhaps I was exposed to some chemicals or toxic materials. Over the years my condition seemed to get slightly worse. I was put on hydroxyurea. The use of hydroxyurea over an extended period of time can lead in some cases to leukemia and other illnesses.

About eight months ago I read your book and I started drinking more water. I drink about 80 ounces a day. Over the years I have also suffered from hypertension and I was under a lot of pressure from my doctor to go on high blood pressure medication. At first my blood pressure was borderline but it seemed to be getting worse. I resisted as long as I could about taking the high blood pressure medication, but I don't think that I could have resisted much longer. I started drinking 80 ounces of water a day eight months ago. Now my blood pressure is totally normal. As a matter of fact, during my last checkup one of the nurses joked that I have the blood pressure of a teenager.

As far as my Polycythemia Vera is concerned there has also been an improvement. As I mentioned above my condition seemed to be getting slightly worse. I started drinking more water eight months ago. Now my condition seems to be improving. Every three months or so I go for a check up and each time they take a sample of my blood for laboratory tests. Among the things they test for, my brother told me, is something called RDW. As best as I can explain what my brother has told me, RDW shows how healthy my cells are, whether they have mutated or not. If they mutate enough, this can lead to leukemia and other medical conditions. This RDW measurement had also been getting slightly worse. The RDW number is now totally normal.

Soon I will ask my doctor whether gradually I can be taken off the medication and rely more on phlebotomy. Both my doctor and my brother have talked about me doing this.

I have described as best as I could both of my medical conditions and how by drinking more water they have both improved significantly. It is a shame that the medical establishment does not take the drinking of larger amounts of water more seriously. I only wish I would have known about all of this many years ago. I do know that I will tell all my friends and relatives about this. I wish I could do much more in helping you promote your theories.

With my best wishes, I remain
Sincerely, Ivan

Allergies; Headache:

I'm doing great!! The pollen in Connecticut has been in the extremely high range for the last month or so. The water and salt have helped me tremendously. Normally, I'd be popping sinus medications every day during this period. I haven't taken any since I've been strictly adhering to the water program. I even gave it a test the other night. I had a long day of driving and delivering milk and other food products to my customers from 8 A.M.–6 P.M. I was exhausted when I got home, muscles were tight, etc. Plus, it was a high pollen day and I had also had a glass of Chardonnay with dinner. Anyway, about 4 A.M., I woke up with a horrible headache. I wasn't sure what caused it, so I took a full glass of water and some salt and went back to bed. I woke up about an hour and a half later and the headache was completely gone, although I was still a bit achy. In the past, I would have taken an antihistamine, but it seemed clear in the book that salt is a natural antihistamine and now "I believe."

One of my customers, an elderly woman, was complaining of an ulcer and acid reflux problem. I told her about the water cure and we figured out her ounces and I said to "give it a try." I saw her a week later and she said it was really helping her out. I gave her a copy of the water book and a few weeks later when I saw her again, she commented that all her symptoms have completely gone.

Thanks for your e-mail, and I'll keep you posted on everyone at my end.
Sincerely, B. T.

Headaches; Joint Pain:

I am writing recently having read your book, *Your Body's Many Cries for Water*. Since following the advice in your book regarding the minimum consumption of water, I have had a complete absence of severe headaches which I had been having daily for about 15 years. I have been taking the maximum dose of Solpadeine tablets (codeine and paracetamol) daily for years, and now have no need of them. I have also ceased drinking tea, coffee and taking chocolate.

The other benefits I notice and others remark on, is my skin and hair have improved, and I have more energy. Previously I also had very sore joints in my feet, and this has been greatly alleviated. All this happened quite quickly after I began drinking only water, and in the quantity your book recommends.
With thanks and warm wishes, A. McG.
Scotland

🌢   🌢   🌢

Migraine Headaches:

For many years I suffered with headaches. I consulted doctors, neurologists, and chiropractors and spent hundreds of dollars for head-scans and x-rays, all to no avail. At times, only my faith in God kept me from wanting to die, as I lay prone on my bed for days on end in pain. No medication would ever stop the pain, it would just seem to run its course and then stop. I could never make any connection between my diet and the headaches, and the only pattern they ever seemed to follow was to always start a couple of hours after a meal.

Then one day a friend told me that he thought my headaches were caused because I never drank enough water. While I knew I didn't actually drink much water, I thought my herbal tea with fruit juices together with lots of fruit amply supplied my liquid requirements. Just three days later I was leafing through a health magazine when an advertisement for your book *Your Body's Many Cries for Water* just seemed to leap out at my eyes. I bought the magazine and sent away for your book.

When it came, I eagerly read and re-read it to learn this new concept about water, and as I saw the errors in my drinking habits I quickly set about righting them. Can anyone, without experiencing it for themselves, really understand what it's like to have usually pain-filled days changed to wonderful painless days when you can do the things you want to do, instead of being "down with a headache"? Oh, such a blessing for which I thank God continually. It has taken months to properly hydrate my body, but now a headache is a now-and-again event instead of the norm. I thank a loving and caring God for leading me step by step to this wonderful truth. He no doubt tried to lead me a lot earlier, but I was too blind to see. I thank you Doctor for your great work and perseverance in bringing this truth to the people.

I lecture to adults at night classes on "Better Food and Eating Habits" and I quickly gave over one of my sessions entirely to the body's needs for water. I have been able to help so many people to better health and much less pain in their lives, with this knowledge. A friend told me he was going into hospital in a few days time for stomach and ulcer treatment. I begged him to cancel this and try the water treatment you recommended. He somewhat reluctantly did and was amazed and thankful to find his pains stop and in time to know the ulcers had healed, without any medication.

Please let me offer my grateful thanks again and pray that the Lord will bless and guide you and your staff as you work for the better health of humanity.
Sincerely, M. B.

Headaches:

A friend of mine recommended I read your book, *Your Body's Many Cries for Water,* and over the past 2–3 months I have been reading it. I have been suffering from headaches for the past 15 years and I had got to the stage that I wasn't sure if the tablets I took were actually giving me the headaches and I was caught up in a vicious cycle. So last September, having read a book called *The Natural Alternative Remedies to HRT,* it suggested giving up tea/coffee. As I have not drunk coffee for years and have drunk tea instead, I thought it would be difficult. However, it has been very easy, and I have been drinking hot water and cold water instead and have given up refined sugars in my diet as well. I never realized how many savory foods contain sugars in various forms until I started reading the labels.

For the first 2 months on this "kick," I got constant headaches, but after perseverance the headaches have disappeared. I only get one and usually I know why—i.e., a glass of wine at lunchtime. But if I drink water, I can usually get rid of the headache without taking any medication. Because I don't get the highs and lows of the blood sugar level, I don't get the cravings for sugar as I did before although I didn't feel I had much sugar to start with in my diet.

Since September I have lost a stone in weight (one stone is 14 pounds of weight). I have always been very fit and active, but now even more so. I feel so much more in control and do not feel the tension of a coiled-up spring ready to snap at any moment as I used to. My friends said at first: "You've lost weight, how did you do it?" I would explain about the headaches and what I did. Now they say: "You look so well, what's the secret?"

So between you and Marilyn Granville, the author of the book I mentioned earlier, I feel a different and a much happier person than I have since 15 years ago when my first child was born. For that, I say a big "Thank You." I am converting my family and friends to the glories of drinking water.
Yours sincerely, Mrs. L. C.

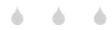

Indigestion; Migraine:

I am an eye surgeon in Columbus, GA, and wish to personally thank you for your series on the body's need for water.

I noticed years ago that by drinking a couple of glasses of water I could alleviate the indigestion that I seem to have been born with. I did nothing with that knowledge, however. I also had migraine headaches for about ten years with often a headache every day. I have noticed that if I drink water until I have to run to the restroom, my headache will go away. I felt that I had eaten something that was a trigger of my headache and that I was flushing this from my body and the combination of a trigger plus dehydration that caused the problem in the first place.

What I am saying is that my observations closely align with yours. Therefore, in listening to your material it immediately opened up my mind to a different way of thinking than what I was used to. I really thank you, and I even thank the Iranian prison system that let you survive and come to America and share this information with us.
Sincerely,
D. Stephen Hollis, M.D.

Migraine:

Thought I'd drop you a note and let you know how increasing my water intake got me off the painkiller Excedrin. After reading your book I hypothesized that water could take its place. I've been taking two to eight tablets per day since college thirty-five years ago and have tried to quit many times. The most I could go was about two or three days before I'd be so sick with a migraine type rebound headache that I'd have to take six or eight tablets a day for several days just to recover from the attempt.

I started two months ago drinking ten or more cups of water a day gradually increasing that amount to sixteen or more cups a day over the first two weeks. During the first week of "rehydration" I still had to take two tablets daily to keep from getting a real banger of a rebound headache. Throughout the second week I was able to get by taking only one tablet a day. Usually by noon a headache would get going but the one tablet seemed to kill it. By the third week I could get by with only 1/2 a tablet. I couldn't believe it and was optimistic about getting off altogether.

On week number four I went without a single tablet, no coffee, tea or pop either. Every time I felt a headache coming on, usually several times a day, I'd drink two or three glasses of water and it would just fade away again. What's more amazing is that during this time life had been busy and stressful as ever. My husband and I are western bronze sculptors, live on a ranch and have five children living at home. We sculpt in clay, make molds of our work, finish our bronze castings and do all our own marketing. I've spent these recent weeks doing an unusually large amount of mold making and wax working. A job that in the past brought on severe eyestrain and sore neck muscles, a sure bet to bring on a three-day debilitating banger of a headache.

This Excedrin/caffeine free streak lasted twelve days before I gave in and took one tablet after an exceptionally long day of tedious mold making. A week later I took a total of three single tablets (one per day for three days). I'm on week number ten now and have been able to keep the headaches at bay with water only for nearly a month. My body has adjusted to the increased water intake. At first I gained a few pounds but now I'm back to what I was a month and a half ago.

I'm so glad my eighty-three-year-young dad, A. N., told me about your book *Your Body's Many Cries for Water*. I am absolutely amazed that it's stopped my headaches. I wanted you to know how good this water treatment was for getting off the Excedrin. In reading about rebound headaches, I've never run across this as a possible painless cure. All these years I drank several glasses of water a day and thought it was enough but I guess I was still dehydrated. Thank you so much for your research and for writing the book.
Sincerely, P. H., Artist

🌢   🌢   🌢

Migraine:

I am a Canadian—I am drinking bottles of water 500 ml. I weigh 135 lbs. and I get the odd migraine and I rechecked your site and discovered that I am not getting enough salt. Thanks for your help. I appreciate it.

Thank God for your site. I've had chronic migraine for 49 years. I fell off a 30-ft balcony when I was four and landed on my head and back. I lived in hell. My teachers, doctors and my parents abused me because 5-year-olds couldn't have migraines. I remember my first migraine; I thought I was going to die.

I had chronic pain that felt like hangovers 6 out of 7 days. I went to doctors, then naturopaths and chiropractors. I had no relief. A friend e-mailed me your site and said why not try it. I was desperate. Your site was an answer to my prayers. I had been drinking water but no salt. When I drank the first bottle of water with the salt, I immediately felt the difference and said "Oh my God." I told my husband, I felt like a new person.

I have been living in Heaven. Life has been glorious. I have tears while I write this. My life is so wonderful since August 2, 2001. Do you know how awesome it is for me to be pain free?? I thought I would die like this.

God bless you for this site. I now have a life. Life is good!!
Thank you so much, N. R.

Migraine; Nausea; Vomiting; Rhinitis; Puffy Eyes:

I have recently read your book *Your Body's Many Cries for Water* and wanted to let you know how many of the things you said relate directly to me. For many years I have suffered from puffy eyes, perennial rhinitis and migraine attacks. By far the most debilitating condition has been migraine, which has seriously affected my personal life and my career as a teacher.

The pain, usually accompanied by nausea, vomiting and flashing lights, has frequently incapacitated me for periods between two and four days with another day or so of feeling generally unwell. My doctor has treated me with Parma, ergotamine, Sandomigran, metoclopramide, Imigran and Prozac with limited success, certainly the pain has been reduced but the actual migraines have continued. My kinesiology therapist recommended that I drink more water and gave me your book to read.

I began drinking about two liters of water every day although I must confess to being skeptical about what this would do for me. Almost immediately I felt somehow different, my eyes looked clearer and the puffy eyelids subsided. I have not had an allergic reaction to anything, which means no wheezing, sore eyes and nose etc., but the biggest difference has been with my migraine attacks. I would like to say that I have had no attacks whatsoever, but that would not be true. I had an attack recently, but instead of lasting for a minimum of two days, it lasted for eight hours, after which I was able to eat and drink normally and resume my everyday activities as though nothing had happened.

This is amazing for me!! My migraine attacks have always been linked to stress, usually occurring when, after a stressful period of worry, I can begin to relax. This most recent attack happened when I had had a great many problems to deal with, over several weeks, and when I could normally expect an attack of four days or so. I intend to continue with your programme and of course, to discuss it with my doctor at our next review meeting. I have already begun to encourage my husband and four sons to drink more water.

Somehow I just know that drinking water, pure water, has changed my health quite immensely, and I am thankful that your book was placed in my hands. I send thoughts of love and peace with gratitude for your work. Sincerely, L. C. M.

◦　◦　◦

Tiredness; Allergies:

Last week I caught part of an interview on the radio about your book, *Your Body's Many Cries for Water*. I went out to purchase it but none of the bookstores had it in stock. I ended up ordering it and finally got it today. The book was outstanding.

While I was waiting for the book I increased my water consumption to no less than two liters a day. I was astonished at how quickly I noticed results in my overall feeling. My energy level increased and I was no longer feeling exhausted at the end of the day. I was previously always tired and feeling as if I wasn't getting enough sleep. I would drink coffee all day just to keep going. I was getting a good eight hours of sleep a night but to no avail; I still felt like I was working on five hours. It didn't matter if I increased my sleep to nine or ten hours, I still felt exhausted. It was getting to the point my wife kept pushing me to go to the doctor. There were also times I would get shaky and felt as if I was going to pass out. I would normally eat some chocolate and it would pass. However, this past week I haven't had that experience. I have even stopped drinking coffee and didn't experience the headaches associated with the caffeine withdrawal. I have even noticed my allergies haven't been bothering me. It is just amazing the change I've experienced over this past week.

I never realized the politics or protection of company dollars behind the health system. I can only hope that you succeed in changing the system. You are a true doctor!
Sincerely, T. E. A.

● ● ●

Headaches; Depression:

Over the past month I have dramatically increased my water consumption. Previously, I never felt thirsty or the urge to drink water. I drank very little water or any other kind of beverage. I had headaches that ranged in severity on an almost daily basis; I would fall asleep very easily and never feel rested. Despite my physical problems, I did not take any drugs for my headaches or for what most doctors would call depression (thankfully!!).

I am very happy to report that since I read your fantastic book *Your Body's Many Cries for Water*, I increased my water intake, I have not experienced any headaches at all and the depressed feeling I get have practically disappeared. I've had no headaches in weeks; I feel more energized and have gotten back into exercising and feeling good. I do get or sense when I'm thirsty and do get the urge to drink more water.

I truly appreciate your efforts in making people understand the importance of water. I tell everyone I know, but have realized that not everyone is willing to listen. It took me a while to come to my senses.

Keep up the good work and please feel free to publish my letter, as you deem necessary.
Sincerely, S. R.

**Migraine; Swelling of Ankle Joint;
Food Allergies:**

What good fortune it was for me the day that I found your book, *Your Body's Many Cries for Water.* I have suffered from migraines for more than 20 years. Just as other people have told you, I also had sought relief from traditional medicine, acupuncture, acupressure, yoga, tai chi, meditation and a variety of special diets. No wonder they didn't work—all the time I was dehydrated.

I followed your guidelines and within a few days my nightly migraines subsided and then disappeared. In addition, other problems have improved for me:

An ankle that had been swollen for 30 years has returned to normal.

Vaginal lubrication has restored. (I am 61 years old and dryness had been a source of considerable discomfort, even pain, for about 40 years.)

Food allergies (particularly wheat) have become less intense. Before drinking water in the amounts you recommend, I could not eat one bite of bread; now I can have two slices of white bread, for the first time in more than 15 years!

As you can imagine, I have been very enthusiastic in spreading your good news. I have told friends, family and my doctor about your wonderful book. I know that it has been discouraging to find such lack of response among the established medical community. Please know that there are many "little people" out here so grateful to you for not losing heart and for continuing your research on our behalf.

Thank you, thank you, and thank you.
Sincerely, C. K.

◊   ◊   ◊

Multiple Sclerosis; Numbness:

My name is F. T. I have M.S. I was diagnosed in April of 2000. The MRI examinations showed the myelin sheath missing and plaque on the brain. My neurologist checked my medical history and said the first time the entire right side of my body went numb and tingly 18 years before was the beginning of my M.S. The first time I had an attack the doctor did all types of tests; he took spinal fluid to have tested but the hospital lost it. The numbness and tingling never completely stopped; you learn to live with it. I was out of work for six months that time. I went twelve years before I had another attack; this time the upper half of my body was affected. The doctor this time did the MRI but nothing showed up in the neck or the brain. I went through a series of nerve conductive tests over the next two years.

I had another attack in April 2000, this time the MRI showed the M.S. in the neck and brain. I had numbness, tingling, pain, slurred speech, lost control of right arm; walking and balance problems, bodily functions slowed down, and was constantly tired.

My doctor put me on Avonex. The medication would only help for three days out of the week. The Avonex started working longer when I started the water and sea salt. I also take cold-pressed flax seed oil, B-complex, lecithin, a good one a day vitamin and potassium. Two and a half months after I started the water cure my numbness and tingling were gone; in the following months my walking and balance improved, my bodily functions returned to normal. In December 2001, I had an appointment with my neurologist. I told him I was going off the Avonex and using just the water cure. He told me he had heard about the water cure. I told him just what you had to take and no alcohol or caffeine; he told me it was a good idea to stop caffeine because it caused certain neurological function to cease in the brain. He put me through all the tests for M.S. and said I was in excellent health. In June of this year, my family doctor is going to redo the MRI to see if my M.S. is completely gone. As an added bonus, I had an enlarged prostate for seven years, my family doctor checked it on my last visit and said it was normal; he did blood work to make sure and everything came back normal.

To deal with the effects of M.S., you need a positive attitude. I haven't felt this good in twenty years.
Thanks to you! F. T.

◦   ◦   ◦

Multiple Sclerosis:

I've had M.S. for about 5 years. My symptoms included being confined to bed for a month, retaining fluid so badly that I couldn't walk & I weighed 175 lbs. Being short, it really showed up on me. I could hardly talk as well. I didn't know what was wrong with me at the time. My husband was concerned and didn't know what to do for me or with me. Another problem was that I had a chronic bladder condition. I have been to numerous doctors and hospitals in Canada, New York City and Pennsylvania. I've had every test that has been written or given to find out what the problem was with my bowels and bladder. I was told that it was a condition that I had to learn to live with and would end up with a colostomy. I am an LPN and I've been a nurse for 44 years.

I've taken all kinds of medications prescribed for me thinking they would help. I was diagnosed for sure with M.S. at Geisinger in Danville last March. They said that I have had M.S. for about 5 years. This last year it got to be severe.

I wasn't really following the Water Cure until it got very severe. My husband tried it and lost 40 lbs. in a month. Even his disposition and nervousness improved. All the medicine that I was taking, I stopped taking. I had seen such an improvement in my intellect, memory, coordination, breathing; upper respiratory problems were gone as well. My bowel and bladder were stagnated, but they now were starting to function the way they should.

I hadn't seen my doctor for a couple of months. When I walked in, he couldn't believe what he saw. "You look wonderful," is what he said to me. He asked what I was doing. I told him that I was on Dr. Batmanghelidj's Water Cure, the water & salt cure! He asked what that was all about. I told him that everyone needs to drink 2 quarts of water daily and add 1/2 tsp. of salt as seasoning on their food. He said evidently it does work because he could see the results in me and said, Marilyn, you have never been in better health. He thinks it is the greatest thing that he has ever heard.

His name is Dr. John Carey. He has an office here in Kingston and another in Dallas. He even tried it himself and has now lost a lot of weight thanks to the Water Cure. He said that this therapy is so simple and unique that it has to get out to the people. He has always been the type of doctor who believes in helping the individual patient and doing whatever is good for the patient; it doesn't matter where it comes from. If it is good for them, he wants them to have it. Something tragic had to happen like Dr. Batmanghelidj being in the prison waiting to be shot to make this discovery. I had to get M.S. to be able to do what I am doing today, which is telling everyone about it. In the Bible, you see salt & water. If we would all eat & drink and do the things like Jesus did when he was on this earth, and we all know he drank water and we all know that he must have eaten salt. We are the salt of the earth, and if it was good enough for Him, it's got to be good enough for us. This has SAVED MY LIFE!

You have my permission to share this letter with any one you want. Sincerely, M. F.

Note: The urgency to bring circulation to deliver water to a vital organ that is getting progressively dehydrated might at times produce microscopic bleeding around the blood vessels to recycle the 94 percent water that is held in blood and its red cells. The process is called vasculitis. It can happen in the stomach, which has been given the label of gastritis. This process often happens in the kidneys, which then become leaky and lose protein and other essential substances in the urine. The renal problem is called nephrosis. It can happen in the lungs, in muscle tissue, in the skin, which is then called purpura. Most tissues are not "bothered" by the solid waste from such microscopic leakage of blood from their blood vessels. The residue is gradually recycled. When this happens in the brain, however, which has a tightly closed circulation, the residue "cakes" and begins to form plaques. Such plaques are seen in Alzheimer's disease, Parkinson's disease, and multiple sclerosis. Nurse M. F.'s first brain scans revealed the widespread presence of plaques, hence confirming the M.S. diagnosis in her case. About a year after her water treatment, her brain scans showed her plaques had cleared up completely, hence her complete recovery from M.S. She has been free of M.S. for a number of years.

   ◊ ◊ ◊

Multiple Sclerosis:

I have had M.S. since 1989. I had periods of partial paralysis and uncomfortable muscle tremors. Until I came down with M.S., I had never drunk water, I lived on coffee, now I drink no coffee and water is my main drink. My girlfriend told me about the water cure in 1995. I thought it was ridiculous. In April of 1996 I went blind in one eye due to M.S. I had no energy and just wanted to sleep. I was on the water cure for a week and a half when I noticed the change. By the end of three weeks my eyesight came back and all other symptoms disappeared and I was filled with an incredible energy that I never had before. My doctor could not believe I got my sight back that fast. He never had that happen before. My doctor didn't even question me as to how I got better. My message for other M.S. sufferers: Try the water cure and do not give up.
Sincerely, B. V. L.

Obesity; Acid Reflux:

For most of my life, I have been overweight. Every family has a "fat child" and this was me. I was told that I was just "big boned" and I should be content with who I was. Then I heard about the water cure through Bob Butts and Connie Giblin. I was skeptical at first, because how could drinking iced tea and cola be such a problem. But I thought that all I really had to lose was my weight. Over a period of a year and a half, I have lost approximately 100 pounds and am no longer the "fat kid" that everyone knew.

But besides losing the weight, I have noticed that acid reflux, which had been a major part of my life, was also now gone; I could now enjoy foods that previously had brought me nothing but sickness. I have also noticed that I also no longer get ear infections that also seemed commonplace and an inevitable problem of life to me at one time.

I also have more energy and feel as if I have become a whole new person. I have energy to do things that would easily wear me out previously.

Thank you Dr. Batman for helping me!
Sincerely, M. C.

◆　　◆　　◆

Obesity; Back Pain:

My wife and I have been following your water program for about 18 months. While we have always been in good health, we are certain that your discovery has no doubt added years and quality to our lives. We have also had two obvious benefits and without any real effort. My wife took off over 30 lbs; and she called it a breeze, especially since she had tried weight-loss programs before, which were always a form of punishment and deprivation. I also took off 15 lbs and found the same. The unique thing about it is that we eat what we want, but aren't nearly as hungry, especially when we always drink a glass or two of water before eating. We can honestly say that you have made losing weight an easy thing to do.

Another thing is that I've had a bad back for nearly thirty years. Any time that I helped out in the warehouse where prolonged lifting was involved, I would limp around for several days while experiencing considerable pain, especially later that same day and the following day. While my back didn't become miraculously healed in a few weeks or a couple of months as I had seen happen to some of my friends, it did become 99% healed in about 15 months and I can do everything that I could do before my injury without pain. To me, that's incredible!

I have passed the information to countless people and found that many had miraculous health benefits in a matter of days. Your discovery has impressed me to the point that my company has told tens of thousands of your discovery by running thousands of newspaper ads (some full page), television ads and radio ads to get the word out. Radio spots alone now number over 400 a month. Many of our customers who were in their early sixties were getting out of their business because of problems of health and age, only to be planning to renew their efforts and some even expanding their business after a few weeks of your program.

Without a doubt, I could write a book on what I've seen. I told everyone who has been helped in any way that I hoped they would feel a moral responsibility to pass this information on to at least ten people who can also gain a considerable health improvement.

This effort has resulted in various interviews and we even helped form a foundation called "The Circle of Light" to help improve the quality of life in northeastern PA in the areas of health, human relations and education. I have spoken to many doctors who have called for information and even interviewed two on a radio program who have stated that they make your water program part of their treatment.

The truth of your work has caught me up with an incredible passion that will not diminish until most of our country accepts what you have done as just common sense. I sincerely thank you for providing me the opportunity of a lifetime in extremely positive public service. Thanks to you Dr. Batmanghelidj, tens of thousands of people in northeastern PA have had their lives improved.

I want you to know how much I appreciate your "Water Cure"; I share this testimonial to help others make healthier lifestyle changes. Your book has changed my life forever! Thank you!
Sincerely yours, Bob Butts

Note: Bob believes in the health miracles hidden in a glass of water so much that his company in the past number of years has spent more than four hundred thousand dollars trying to educate the people in north-eastern Pennsylvania that they should consider water as a natural medication in most health problems. He even put up a fifty-thousand-dollar reward for children with asthma who tried the water cure and did not get rid of their asthma. Many newspapers and radio programs announced the program. It was amazing that no one came forward to claim their share of the reward money, but countless number of people came forward and told him their asthma was cured because of his announcement. He is taking a truly dedicated and sincere responsibility for educating people in his region of the country that for most of their health problems, they are in effect thirsty and indeed not sick. He now has an army of followers. He has reached and saved thousands of people from the agony of their health problems. God bless him.

Weight Loss:

In August of 1995, at age fifty, I found myself approaching 400 pounds. I swore to myself I would never hit 400. Life became a very painful experience. Every move I made was a painful episode as I struggled to survive. I also began having arthritic pains in my joints; so much that just shaking someone's hand was an unbelievably painful experience. Topping it off was a slipped disc in my back, so you can imagine just getting out of bed was a major effort.

I began getting depressed and irritated. I would find more things wrong than right with others and myself. At that point, I hit my pain threshold and that's when I came across a radio program with your message on wellness with water. Thank God for hearing this message. I heard about your book on that program and decided to read it. After reading it I decided to make some drastic changes in my life, which I did. My weight leveled off at 399 pounds. Then it started dropping. The more I drank water and ate salt, the better I felt and the better I looked. I lost a total of 156 pounds and reduced 14 pant sizes. And I did this by drinking the amount of water you recommend, using table salt and walking.

Since losing the weight, I no longer have the stress on my joints and my back feels great. If you told me a year ago that I could feel this great, I would have said you're crazy, but it worked and I am living proof. I find myself telling everyone I can about your book and the greatest health discovery in history! I hope this letter will help others to try your cure, water and salt. It makes so much sense and it's so simple. I hope people will just try it for their own health's sake instead of becoming addicted to every medicine out there.

Thank you very much for your discovery.
Sincerely, L. D.

◊   ◊   ◊

Panic Attacks; Asthma:

Imagine having to sleep in an upright position for almost a year, struggling for each breath and suffering from countless asthma and panic attacks nightly! On March 27, 1993, I was hospitalized with a severe asthma attack and developed bronchial pneumonia! My blood gases registered 40 and I was in a life-threatening situation!

After my release from the hospital, I was placed on large doses of theophylline and prednisone. My weight skyrocketed and the medication caused me to become hostile and disoriented. I really didn't want to live! Then, a wonderful friend gave me a flyer on Dr. Batmanghelidj's book *Your Body's Many Cries for Water!* I quickly mailed a check and a letter to the doctor, pleading for a fast delivery! To my complete surprise, he called me personally and started helping me by telephone to get off the medication, which was inappropriate for my condition at this time, and asked me to drink at least three liters of water a day and use a small amount of salt. He also asked me to walk in an indoor shopping mall for 15 minutes a day. I can now walk for 30 minutes a day and my breathing is 100% better!

As of this date, October 31, 1994, I am no longer on any medication for asthma! I have not used an inhaler or medication of any sort for more than five months! When I start any sort of mild wheezing, I just drink a glass of water and take a little salt and I'm fine!

And guess what???? All the wonderful water and walking has made me lose 35 lbs. I'm back to my desired weight and I look young, vibrant and healthy again!

There are millions of Americans out there who need to get the message. They suffer from AIDS, asthma, arthritis and chronic fatigue syndrome, etc. Everyone in America could benefit from reading Dr. Batmanghelidj's books!
Very sincerely, P. P.

**Blood Pressure; Weight Loss;
Allergies; Back Pain:**

I again wish to thank you for your kindness in helping my wife and me to better appreciate the importance of water to our health.

We feel the conscious increase in our water consumption contributed greatly to our weight loss—a weight loss that had been urged upon both of us by our respective physicians for years. My loss of approximately 45 pounds has resulted in such a lowering of my blood pressure. My wife's weight loss has alleviated the discomfort she has experienced for years with her back. In addition, she believes the weight loss has reduced her discomfort and problems with her allergies.
With best wishes, I remain
Sincerely, E. M. P.

Excess Weight; Diabetic:

On February 12 my doctor called me with the results of my blood test and informed me that I had diabetes type-2, as my Hemoglobin ALC was 7.3 and I weighed 348lbs. The next day I started the water cure, drinking 5 quarts of water and adding 1 tsp. of salt to my food. I just had my latest blood test on July 2nd, and here are the results.

Date	02/12/02	07/02/02
Weight	348	296
Tryglycerides	288	138
Cholesterol	247	189
Glucose	191	108
Hemoglobin ALC	7.3	5.4

I wasn't able to exercise during this time due to a bad back. So these results were achieved through the water and salt program. I eat all the normal foods. I am now starting to introduce an exercise routine using Dr. B.'s book for backs and can't wait to see the results. I would have never been able to get to this point without the water and salt and am eternally grateful to you and Dr. B. I now tell everyone I know now about the water cure. Many thanks.
Thank you, J. K.

💧   💧   💧

Weight Loss; Blood Pressure:

It is a pleasure to sit down and chronicle the effects that this lifestyle change has meant to me both professionally and personally. On a professional basis, I was asked by AWANE Executive Director to listen to a tape called *Your Body's Many Cries for Water.*

The tape immediately created a desire for me to adopt its suggestions. I began this lifestyle change on June 10 and began drinking much more water daily. Since that start date, I have

- Lost 46 lbs
- Blood pressure at normal—no meds needed
- Skin elasticity has returned
- Athlete's foot cured
- Asthma medication reduced
- Pain in lower back eliminated
- Foot pain eliminated
- Diabetes symptoms gone

I have eliminated the diuretics mentioned in the book and have lost a taste or craving for those products.

Yours truly, J. R.

◊ ◊ ◊

Sleep Disorder; Headaches;
Joint Pain; Irritable and Intolerant:

Would like to thank you for your hard work in getting the information about water out to the public. I have had such amazing results in just two weeks. I was drinking four Cokes a day and maybe 16 to 32 ounces of water and lots of chocolate. Everyone has been begging me to stop the Cokes but it didn't hit home until I heard your program on the Art Bell show.

I started on 80 ounces of water and 1/4-teaspoon salt the next day. I cut down to only two Cokes a day and I'm weaning off of them slowly because I'm so addicted. I was very nervous and irritated over the least thing that would happen. Seemed like I was headed for a nervous breakdown because of stress in my life. I couldn't sleep soundly and all of my joints were aching. Also, I felt my heart was very strained whenever I would walk up steps or exert myself; I would be out of breath. I had sinus headaches and took two Sine-Aids every day, which I'm sure didn't help. My daughter just graduated from college and moved back home and I couldn't handle living with someone.

My family and friends have been very concerned because I seemed to be losing self-control. When I started the water and salt I couldn't

believe the results. I feel laid back and calm like I used to be. I'm getting along great with my family and friends and they have commented
on my changes and they have started the water also!! I have lost about
five pounds without dieting and I feel a lot more energy. Not the spurts
of energy I used to feel, but I'm not dead tired when I get off work at
11:45 P.M. Have a little reserve tank left. But, when I am tired I can
now sleep instead of feeling like my mind will not stop racing. I used to
never feel thirsty, just wanted a lift. Now, I am thirsty and craving the
water and have always had to force myself to drink water before. I will
keep going and get off of the two Cokes and Sine-Aid and probably do
even better. I ordered your tape on M.S. to pass on to three friends who
have the disease. I will let you know what I hear back from them.
Sincerely, M. L.

Obesity:

In November of 2000, I weighed 525 lbs. Now, January of 2003, I weigh
225 lbs. Here is how I did it.

My story is simple. For thirty-two years of my life I continued to eat all
the wrong foods and drink every unhealthy drink imaginable. My life
for thirty-two years was a happy one. I had lots of friends, good jobs and
a wonderful, but sickly mother. I got around pretty well for someone of
my size. I was active, playing sports and competing in karate, all such
activities that would promote a healthy lifestyle or weight loss. I however ate everything that was bad for you in large amounts, at the wrong
times and would follow it up by drinking liters of soda or alcohol.

I look back now and could honestly say without any reservation that
there were times of up to a month that I would not have any water.
Water never tasted good to me, and as far as could remember, it would
always give me a stomachache. Maybe it did. Maybe it was psychological, because I really didn't need or want to drink water. I loved soda
and could easily sit and drink a two-liter bottle with one meal. One
meal could be a large pizza with everything and chicken wings, 10:30 at
night. I could recall two to three times a week I would order from a

local pizza place a large cheese steak with extra cheese and a meatball with extra cheese and eat both with a two-liter soda, again very late at night. The times I remember eating the most was when I was alone at night or just getting home from work late at night, not tired and would eat. Even at the times when I wasn't really hungry. It became routine for me to do this regularly.

My mornings weren't the best either. I made daily stops to the local McDonald's on my way to work to order two to three breakfast sandwiches and again my favorite soda. Looking back now I realized this routine went on for years to the point I couldn't say honestly when I started this massive destruction of my body. It didn't help to have a few friends who were also big people who ate a lot. My friends and I would regularly hit every buffet in the city. It got to the point where we were recognized and our names called out like Norm on "Cheers." Not something to be proud of. Earlier on I stated I was a very happy person and had many wonderful friends. However I was very lonely, I had no one to share myself with.

Just about all of my friends were married, in love and had beautiful companions to come home to. Everything I always wanted for myself but was not realistic at my size. Losing weight was not believable to me. My mother was very ill, in and out of the hospital multiple times with lung disease. A few times she almost didn't make it. I was very scared and again found another excuse to eat and eat a lot. My mother did eventually get a little better and didn't need me there all the time.

In November of 2000, at the age of thirty, I started seriously considering stomach stapling to help me lose weight, if I wanted to honestly live. At that weight the chances of living much longer wouldn't be too good. I was feeling the stress of my massive weight on all my joints was getting ill more often and was hospitalized multiple times with deep vein thrombosis. I was very scared and very alone. I knew it was time to get serious about losing weight or die. I guess you're wondering how much I weighed. I weighed a whopping 525 lbs. I wore a six-extra-large shirt and had a waist line of seventy-two. On January 21st of 2001, I started my very long journey to a new life.

I had a very good friend who pushed me nightly for three months straight to go with him to the gym and eat the right foods at the right times. Most importantly drink a lot of water. I mean a lot of water. I hated water, but I knew if I really wanted to lose weight I needed to do the right thing and stop playing games. At this time for the first time in my life I was confident about myself and knew I had it in me to lose any amount of weight I needed to. I met a wonderful woman at about the same time I began my journey to become healthy and hopefully thin. My friend pushed me harder and was always there for me not to give up. I made up my mind to give up all liquids besides water and a popular diet drink. It helped me a lot. I would wake up every morning and have a diet drink and drink a 24 oz glass of water. I would drink three more 24 oz glasses of water before lunch, have another diet drink and continue with my regimen of water until dinner. I would drink a 24 oz glass of water leading up to dinner to help me feel full and not want to eat as much.

I became very drastic with my eating habits and food. I would never eat past six o'clock at night and again only water to help me feel full. Let me tell you I went to the bathroom all the time. I gave up all breads, pasta, and potatoes, everything that had carbohydrate in it. Most importantly I gave up all soda, even diet decaffeinated. My carbohydrate intake was about twenty grams a day and my saturated fat intake was about two to three grams a day. I know you're saying that your body needs fat to survive. You are absolutely right. I was prepared during my weight loss in what is healthy and what isn't while dieting. I read and read multiple books on vitamins and supplements to make sure I wasn't depriving my body of what it needed. I also saw a doctor regularly. I began taking daily essential fatty acids in pill form along with a multi vitamin, a vitamin B complex 150, calcium, vitamin C and a sublingual vitamin B12. All of which I learned help with energy metabolism and the breakdown of stored fat, carbohydrates and sugar.

A great person, and now great friend, who owned a local fitness store, broke it down for me honestly and helped me with my supplement regiment. My nightly cardiovascular and weight routine began to get easier as I began losing weight fast. I was almost losing a pound of weight a day. People were getting worried but I remained true to eating the right foods and drinking the huge amounts of water. My doctor continued to monitor me and was not too concerned with my rapid weight loss. My blood pressure was getting better along with my resting heart rate lowering and, thank God, no problems with sugar diabetes.

I guess you are wondering what I was eating. Well I was eating large amounts of canned tuna and canned chicken. Protein, protein, and protein, as much as I could get, lots of salad with no dressing, turkey burgers, vegetable burgers and again lots and lots of chicken and tuna. Yes I was sick of eating the same thing all the time. However, I kept reminding myself the diet and exercise was working and I was losing weight. I encouraged myself to believe that pasta, pizza, soda, cheeseburgers and other junk weren't more important to me than my life. Oh yes, let me tell you of the wonderful woman I mentioned briefly earlier on. I continued to see her and her two beautiful boys. This was more motivation to continue than anything anyone could imagine. I was in love and most importantly someone was in love with me. Yes, she fell in love with the fat me, which makes her even more special to me.

As the months went on I continued ever diligently on my exercise and water regimen. I never felt sick and I never again had any problems with the veins in my legs. People were beginning to notice the change that was occurring. It was getting drastic. My waistline was falling along with my shirt size. In case you forgot I weighed 525 lbs. At the end of the first year of my dieting, January 21st 2002, I weighed 250 lbs. I lost 275 lbs working very hard with friends and on my own. My current weight today, as of the New Year 2003, is 225 lbs. I found that this is a very good weight for me. I have put on good muscle and shrunk down to a large shirt and a 38 waist comfortably. I do have a lot of skin, but hope to eventually get surgery to have it removed. A lot of skin from a lot of fat is a good trade off to me.

Keeping the weight off is easy to me now that I have tons of energy, can get around and running on the treadmill up to three miles at a time surely helps a lot. Yes I currently eat all the foods I used to eat. Cheeseburgers, pizza, pasta, potatoes and occasionally some candy. It's all about one word, moderation. Never ever again I will drink soda. Water. . . . Water . . . . . Water . . . (Ok, diet green tea and diet drinks.)

Is all the weight loss real to me? I still don't believe it sometimes. When I look into a mirror, there are times I don't believe it's me.

The first real time I knew I was actually thin and not fat is when I walked in front of a group of little kids going to school. None of them stared at me, or laughed, or made a fat comment. I had just passed the little kids' test. During my years of being fat I knew that kids were the toughest and most honest. My life today is everything I had dreamed about. Well it's no longer a dream. I have married the woman I spoke about and became a father to her two wonderful boys. Today we live a beautiful life in a beautiful home with a very happy and healthy life. If there is anything I can say to help anyone who reads this story: it is to never give up. Dreams can be reality. Follow good advice and do it for you. There is a famous quote that I kept in my wallet through my dieting and it still remains there today. Martin Luther King stated, "We must accept finite difficulties, but we must never lose infinite hope." I HAVEN'T AND NEVER WILL! D. C.

Note: D. C. lives in northeastern Pennsylvania—Bob Butt's area of the country—where a lot is known about the healing powers of water, including its effectiveness in weight-loss programs.

Bee Sting:

I am a seventy-six-year-old retired teacher and former combat Marine (WWII & Korea). Our gated community has a swimming pool and spa near our residence. We use them almost daily.

A year ago, while climbing out of the pool, I grasped the rail to help myself climb up the stairs. I felt a sharp pain in the palm of my hand and immediately recognized a bee falling off my hand. (When I was a child I had an allergy regarding bee stings but had not been bothered by the problem for many years.) Soon, my hand began to swell and the pain increased severely. I recalled a comment I heard an M.D. make on a recent TV program about the necessity to drink lots of water in order to flood the system and wash toxins out of the body. I quickly determined to cooperate with my own need. I left the pool area and headed for home.

At home I chug-a-lugged a 12-ounce glass of water. Every 15 minutes I chug-a-lugged another full glass of water. An hour and a half later I had drunk six 12-ounce glasses of water—and at that time the pain ceased suddenly and the swelling went down. It is a lesson I will never ever forget.

Now, I drink five or six glasses of water a day—whether I have a problem or not. Can water be patented? HA!
Best regards, J. B.

Allergies; Headaches:

Thank you for being on the *Sightings* program some time back. I've increased my water uptake since then and have been feeling so much better. I have more energy and while I've had one cold it didn't last long and it didn't go into bronchitis as it usually does. It was just one rather than a number. My doctor told me to lose weight and I have found that it is a lot easier to do so if I'm drinking water most of the day.

I live in the Ohio River valley and we have a lot of allergies, however this summer, I haven't had any problems. My head is clear and have had no headaches. I guess the best answers are the obvious ones. Thank you and God bless you, E. O.

Acne; Skin:

I have been following your recommendations in your book, *Your Body's Many Cries for Water,* for the past two weeks, and would like to share my observations with you. The first thing I noticed was that my skin, even the "hard" skin on my feet, felt softer. I looked in the mirror and noticed the lines that had begun to circle my neck—I am fast approaching 40—have faded a lot; the same with the lines at the corners of my mouth, my frown lines, and the "furrows" in my forehead. Was I happy!

But more importantly, the acne I have endured for most of my life, since I was 12, has cleared approximately 70% and I expect continued improvement as I continue on this program. I have seen a number of dermatologists, taken far too many antibiotics for my body's own good; I have been put on Retin-A therapy along with Accutane that "dried up" my oil glands, which indeed eliminated the acne, but made my skin break out in a horrible rash that made me look like an alligator-woman, not to mention the possibility of liver damage. I was so frightened. I stopped taking it at once, and 6 months later, my acne was back in full force. Finally I decided it was better to just live with the acne than keep putting myself through all of that. I am sure you know acne has a terrible effect on a person's self-esteem and confidence. I wish I had had your book when I was 12! My life might have been quite different. Well, better late than never! I can never thank you enough.

Dr. Batmanghelidj, thank you again for your wonderful book. It has made a real difference in my life. May God bless you.
Sincerely, T. C. H.

$$\delta \quad \delta \quad \delta$$

Heartburn; Kidney Stone:

Thank you for standing up for the simple. I've really enjoyed reading your book (many times) and thought it was about time I wrote you of my experiences.

I'm 37 years old. Before reading your book I was told to increase my water intake by my doctor. I had all the symptoms of a urinary tract infection; but urinalysis didn't show anything but highly concentrated urine.

I began drinking a gallon-plus of water daily while waiting for further tests. We had to go on a two-week trip during which time pain while urinating became very extreme. I also had some very mild kidney cramps. When we got home, I passed what the doctor said was a very large kidney stone, and instantly felt like a new man! Also, for the past 15 years I've been hooked on antacids to control daily heartburn— since increasing my water intake, I don't need them anymore.

During this period, I've also broken a 20-year addiction to cigarettes. I've tried many times before but this time was easier, the water. Thank you, D. L.

Swelling; Weight Loss:

Thank you for forwarding the information regarding AIDS as a metabolic disorder from the *Science in Medicine Simplified Journal.* During the past year I have experienced many stressful life situations and have decided to look more seriously at my health and the care of my body. I have also started a master's degree in wellness science to further my knowledge for myself and for sharing with others. One of the most interesting and important subjects and one of your favorites is water along with exercise and proper protein intake.

As I progress through my studies and begin to incorporate this new info and knowledge, I am finding a general overall increased well-being. I have more energy, stamina, sleep better, feel more peaceful, lost weight and am beginning to see a difference in the edema swelling in my legs.

I am very appreciative for all that you share and I am daily sharing with others the importance of water and the other information that you so adequately shared in your book and related references.

Thank you kindly and you can rest assured that I am doing my utmost in educating the public about the importance of water. Warmest regards, J. P.

Weight Loss; Headache; Heartburn;
Blood Pressure; Back Pain; Muscle Cramps;
Kidney Function:

I want to thank you for writing the books *Your Body's Many Cries for Water*, and *The ABC of Asthma, Allergies and Lupus*. Because of these books, I am a living testimonial to the value of water and salt. I had a kidney transplant five years ago and my health was failing until August 22, 2002, when a customer, Mr. James Bolen, took one look at me and told me I was dehydrated. He asked me to drink two glasses of water and put a little salt on my tongue. I was reluctant at first but he convinced me to try it. In five minutes I didn't feel sick anymore. My headache was gone and I had more energy. I felt like a new person.

Mr. Bolen told me to stop all caffeine, no tea or coffee, soda or chocolate. I asked why? He told me he would send me your books to read and fax me a list of suggested foods to eat and recommended the water and salt program. I was told by my doctor to stay away from salt. My doctor even had me on a water pill. Mr. Bolen told me he was only a truck driver but had read your books many times. He recommended I stop the water pill and start the water and salt program gradually, making sure to measure the amount of water my kidney was putting out. It had to equal input or stop the program immediately. I thanked Mr. Bolen for his time and knowledge but was very reluctant to follow his advice since it was against my doctor's orders. Next evening I went to the hospital for two days only to receive three bottles of saline solution. I was taken off my water pill and sent home. At home, I found out that Mr. Bolen had since faxed me some more information about the "Water Cure" and also received a copy of your books. I started reading them and decided to try the program in earnest.

Since I started, I haven't experienced any heartburn, headaches and my blood pressure is back to normal. I feel more energized, sleep much better, eat less food and have lost a whopping 40 lbs to date! My back pain is gone and no more muscle cramps!! My last checkup was perfect and my doctor was very impressed with my health and weight loss and it feels like my own kidneys are starting to gradually function.

It is so simple but we are so blind from commercialization. I am very grateful to God for sending Jim Bolen to my place of work that day and Dr. Batmanghelidj's books and research. May God bless you both and keep up the good work.
Sincerely, A. C. B.

Blood Pressure; Diverticulitis; Cholesterol; Constipation:

Being in my 69th year, high blood pressure, high cholesterol and diverticulitis have for years spurred me to be more thoughtful of diet, exercise, and what I permit my thinking to include. I would have been on drugs 10 years ago, except for having chosen the drug-free route. Having tried several times over the years to drink more water, I have not been able to stick with 8 glasses a day until February this year, when a friend gave me a copy of your book.

Although I still take herbal-fiber-blend, which has been a Godsend for me, I realized after two weeks of drinking 6–8 glasses of water daily that my bowel movements have never been as good as they are now. Abdominal pains, which periodically have caused me to faint while on the toilet, have been totally absent, since my having become consistent with 8 glasses of water daily.

Knowing that you credit our Creator with what appears to be your own doing, multiplies my faith and trust that it is possible to put the credit where it belongs. Circulating complimentary copies of your book, *Your Body's Many Cries for Water*, makes me feel good. My method of doing so at this time is to mail or hand out copies of the book review requesting that they let me know if they would like a complimentary copy of the book. Response has been good. About 20% requests copy of the book, one of whom I am delighted to say is my doctor. Hopefully I am not breaking any copyright law by making photo-copies of the review "Borderland Volume—First Quarter 1997." I trust you will advise if I am. Seeing infinite possibilities for the health-care-related paradigm shift of which you speak, I remain with best wishes and gratitude.
Sincerely, B. D.

Allergies; Heartburn:

Thank you for your response. I am a Registered Nurse. I have been trained to think in terms of drugs for a long time. Drug reps are frequent visitors and educators with CEU info. I have also for over 10 years had to take Zantac, Prilosec, Prevacid, Maalox, and Gaviscon on a daily basis. I read the *ABC of Asthma, Allergies, and Lupus* and have to admit I was very skeptical. However, the thing that intrigued me was that there couldn't possibly be any monetary reason to shift someone into a water regimen.

There is just no money in it. I also was getting a bit desperate, since, in spite of everything, the medication wasn't working. My doctor was talking of a surgery that would cut nerves in my stomach to reduce the acid production. I am not thrilled with this type of permanent mutilation. I decided to give water a try. It has been nearly two weeks since I decided to give it a try. I have not had any drugs since. As a bonus, my fall allergies have gone away. I am absolutely stunned. I also am sharing it with my patients. I also used to find it very difficult to stick to a diet and have had a lot of trouble losing weight. Not any more. I have lost 5 pounds in 10 days and feel it much easier to say no to snacks. I just wish more people knew about this.
Sincerely, D. B.

Alcohol Addiction; Weight Loss:

My father introduced me to your water discoveries at a very critical time for me and my infant son. I am 35 years old and had been an alcoholic since my twenties. As with most people so afflicted, my personal relationships were rocky and impermanent, and I had a broken marriage behind me. I had also just reached the end of a follow-on relationship, in a fashion that was both shocking and stressful, since I was without resources to continue my life in a city strange to me. I got into AA determined to prevent any repetition of my agonies.

At this point, my father gave me your book and urged me to act on its content with full resolve. I did so, grasping at what I saw as an unexpected deliverance—like the hand of God. I was gratified to discover the power of water to still the cravings of an alcoholic. Soon I realized that alcoholism was really a *THIRST SIGNAL* that I was habituated to respond to with alcohol, which is a powerful dehydrating agent. One became like a dog chasing its own tail. Dehydration through alcohol is self-perpetuating, unless the thirst sensations are answered with water.

Persevering with adequate daily water intake, and eliminating dehydrating caffeinated drinks, I found myself able to deal effectively with my personal locational crisis. I was able to get my belongings and furniture together, rent a truck, load it, and drove my son and myself back to California from Las Vegas. My former alcoholic self could not have done this. I resettled myself in California, went back successfully into my work as a beautician, and buckled down to raising my son.

Of course I still have normal problems like everyone else, but alcohol is not one of them. Water has lifted this curse from my life. As I write, I have been ten months "dry" and I have been able to reorganize my life rationally. Adequate daily water intake is the bedrock on which to rebuild a life deranged by alcohol, and to help others do the same. There are other benefits that will have great appeal to all alcoholic women in particular.

As an alcoholic, I had begun to lose my youthful looks. Steady self-poisoning and dehydration with alcohol dulled and aged my complexion. In recent years, my weight had steadily increased for the reasons you outline so clearly in your book. I began to look puffy and pallid. Therefore I was elated—absolutely "stoked"—when rehydration caused my excess weight to just disappear. I could not believe it, nor could my friends, as I regained the perfect figure I had enjoyed as a young woman. I did not have to "sweat" this, it just happened! My complexion began to change back to a wonderful, youthful glow that everyone remarks on, which has delighted my father. My regained radiance is a big asset in my professional work as a beautician. The weight loss and adequate daily water intake invigorated my whole being. I began running on what you call "hydro-electric power," in your book.

With these changes came an overall renewal of life and outlook. I continue to help others through AA. I began attracting life-positive gents of purpose and substance, instead of the lesser fellows who would tolerate an alcoholic woman. Church attendance brought me comfort, and I wanted to attend. I plan and work for an ever-improving life. Reviewing my past from my normalized perspective, I apologized to my father for my many years of outrages, and for the suffering I had caused him because of his love for me. Dad had almost given up on me, but his provision of your book was decisive in my redemption.

My father tells everyone that you are one of the greatest physicians in the history of the world. I think he is right. Thank you Dr. Batmanghelidj, for all you have done, not only for me with my turn-around in life, but also for all mankind.
Very sincerely yours, D. R. E.

Salt Prevents Nausea:

I have always been a water drinker, and sometimes I've been made fun of for it, but I didn't always drink 8–10 glasses a day. When I was growing up, the other kids would drink pop almost every day, but I was allowed to only on occasion. Back in the late 50s I started caring for older folk that were to be on salt-free diets. Thinking it would be better for me, I went on one too. In November of 1993 I got your book *Your Body's Many Cries for Water*, and I started to drink at least 10 glasses of water a day. Your suggestion of drinking two glasses at a time helps. A month later I was nauseated with emesis. Then I started to put one-quarter teaspoon of salt in the water each day, and I must say I noticed a great improvement in how I feel.

It has been over five years since I had a cold. Thank you for your efforts.
Healthfully yours, I. J. C.

Eczema:

Hi, I am currently using the water cure to speed up weight loss. It was suggested on a low-carb bulletin board for friends of the Atkins way of eating. Just wanted you to know that right now I don't even care if it helps with weight loss, I feel so much better after only 6 days on water cure. My stress-related eczema is clearing up; my skin feels good and even my hair feels great. A lot of the other Atkins friends are reporting benefits from water cure along with weight loss.
Thanks for listening, Pamela.

Headaches; Tinnitus:

I already told you how my headaches disappeared by drinking more water. I can hardly feel my heartbeat and my color is better. The vein I could see on my left leg is disappearing and also on my right leg. The discomfort on the left side of my chest is all but gone. I am working on my swelling eyelids and tinnitus. It has been four months since I started more water. I am 52 years old, and it seems to me there is so much money spent on medications for problems water would cure.
Sincerely, D. P.

P.S. Thanks for writing the book.

Narcolepsy:

My name is C. J. and I was diagnosed with narcolepsy (a neurological sleep disorder) over 15 years ago. I have implemented the "water cure" as of a month ago and have been able to eliminate my medication (a powerful CNS). Halleluiah!!

Just thought I would share the good news with others.
Sincerely, C. J.

Intestinal Obstruction; Acid Reflux:

Your book on dehydration, *Your Body's Many Cries for Water*, has significantly changed my life. I can't thank you enough for all your exhaustive research and the endless hours you must have spent compiling your data.

My name is D. S. and I am a 53-year-old building contractor. I have always drunk plenty of soda, coffee, tea and some beer. I mistakenly thought I was getting enough water via these beverages. Two years ago I became ill with high fevers and gastric esophageal reflux disease. At night my condition worsened and eventually I was hospitalized. I was diagnosed with an ileo-intestinal blockage. My condition was further compromised by aspiration pneumonia, second to vomiting. And to make matters worse I developed a Guillian-Barré syndrome of ascending neuropathy due to the effect this intestinal problem created with my immune system. May 1997 the surgical procedure "ileo-jejunoscopy" was performed to relieve the bowel obstruction. My hospital stay lasted two weeks due to the pneumonia and my compromised condition. I had lost a tremendous amount of body weight in the course of my illness.

I began having similar symptoms of gastric reflux, constant diarrhea, and vomiting during March of this year. I tried a medicine course of Pepcid, Zantac, Maalox and Prilosec. I also began losing weight, suffered from leg cramps at night, and even had problems with urinary incontinence. My Dr. sent me for an upper and lower GI and diagnosed me with another partial bowel obstruction—of course I was scheduled for surgery. One week before surgery a friend insisted that I read your book. Dr. Batmanghelidj, I sat down and read your book that first night—and a light went on in my head. I drank four glasses of water, sips at a time until completion. That night I slept without reflux or leg cramps. I then continued with 8 to 10 glasses a day; and by the 3rd day, my abdominal cramping and diarrhea had completely stopped. I was able to eat normal meals without discomfort. By the 5th day I had started gaining weight and strength. On the 6th day, I called my surgeon and told him to take me off the surgical schedule.

Dr., I am feeling much better now than I have in several years, and to think that all I needed was WATER. I now know I was suffering from internal dehydration and not a single physician, surgeon, or specialist had a clue.

Thank you again and again for caring and for your dedication. Should you ever be in the Philadelphia area and need a live testimony, I would avail myself to further your cause.
Warmest regards, D. S. S.

⬦   ⬦   ⬦

Headaches; Loss of Memory:

I just finished your book on water, and am responding to your call for testimonials.

I am 39 years old. For all my life I have suffered from one problem or another: mental, emotional, and on occasion physical. I am overweight and eat poorly; I have been anorexic, bulimic, suicidal and just about anything else you can think of.

I have suffered allergies and sinus problems for 20 years. Daily headaches for the last eight years. About six years ago I noticed an alarming increase in memory problems, severe enough that I visited my family physician, concerned I was experiencing "early onset Alzheimer's." His diagnosis? The brain can only hold so much information and it must release some to take in new. Lucky for me he didn't prescribe any new medication; I was already on five or six different medications. Now my headaches—I started with Advil, Tylenol or Excedrin. I reached the point where I was taking 7–8 pills as much as 2–3 times daily. To counter the eating of my stomach I was taking them with chocolate milk. Then I found 800 mg prescription Tylenol or rather ibuprofen. I was back to only one pill until I had to start increasing it by Nov. 1999. I was taking 2–3 of those as much as four times a day. I might add at this time my choice of liquid every day for the last 20 years has been Diet Pepsi. I never drank water!!

April 17, 2000, I began drinking water, a minimum of 1/2 a gallon per day up to a gallon when I could. Within 2 days I lost my desire for Diet

Pepsi, within a week my headaches stopped completely. I have been off all my medications completely. In one month I have experienced a complete change in mood, depression, have not had any sinus problems and only one very slight headache. Needless to say my life has changed, radically improved by WATER!! My only problem on two occasions was unexplained episodes of dizziness that have now been explained by your chapter on salt.

I hope never to swallow another pill in my life. Thank you.
Kindest Regards, V. H.

Ascites:

A couple of years ago I read your book *Your Body's Many Cries for Water* and I wrote to you asking how I could drink so much water and not swell up? (I explained to you about my liver disorder of cavernous transformation of the portal vein with portal hypertension and my trouble with ascites and swelling of my abdomen from time to time.) You responded personally and told me how to drink the water and avoid this problem. I am happy to report that to my surprise my body did get acclimated to the extra water and it now swells up when I don't drink it. I just wanted to let you know you were correct and I later came across the use of other types of water therapy as a cure for ascites and other maladies in the book *Honey, Mud, Maggots and Other Medical Marvels* by Robert Root-Bernstein.
Best Regards, T. M. R.

Note: Ascites is a condition in which the abdomen becomes water-logged from inside and builds up "an ocean" around the organs in the abdominal cavity. You hear it splashing when the body moves. It occurs with severe liver damage from liver infections, alcoholic fibrosis of the liver, or secondary growths of cancer in its terminal stages. It is my opinion that ascites could also occur with severe edema of dehydration, when the body is in overdrive to retain water for use in its reverse-osmosis program of filtering and injecting load-free water into vital cells. Drinking clear and clean water by itself will always siphon out stagnant edema, which is water that contains much dissolved materials and toxins.

◊   ◊   ◊

Dehydration:

In 1991 I felt strangely sick in bed and I was ambulanced to an army emergency room. The ambulance attendant said she couldn't find a prominent vein to start an IV, as they were all flat. Doctors in the emergency room also couldn't start an IV of glucose. I stayed there for 12 hours and never needed to urinate. I drank 2–3 pitchers of water and was able to ambulate and walk out feeling much improved. Later I learned about the book titled *Your Body's Many Cries for Water.* It made sense to me.

I started on the water treatment protocol. I am an octogenarian who has been dehydrated most of my life unknowingly to me. I heartily recommend Dr. Batman's water regime. It has helped me stay healthy during my "declining" years and I am declining drugs, antibiotics, flu shots, pain pills and over-the-counter stuff, and I am feeling fine. Folks say I look younger than my 83 calendar years.
Aloha, M. R.

◊   ◊   ◊

Constipation:

Thanks for this website. I appreciate the good sense and well-documented scientific sources of this revelation. I recently experienced a bladder infection and significantly increased my water consumption. Constipation caused by my medication completely went away, and I feel better than ever. Why did my doctor not advise me to drink sufficient water when I was seriously constipated and chronically uncomfortable? This is information learned in grade school health classes; I would think that a physician could simply remind me to drink water!! I also have relapsing-remitting M.S. and hope that this new habit can keep me

healthy. It makes me wonder if my years of alcohol abuse and subsequent dehydration may have brought on this condition. I cannot thank you enough for your good sense and educated endorsement of such a simple cure. Thank you also for this web site—I'm so glad that I was led to it!!
E-mail message sent to www.watercure.com

Sleep:

I want to express my deepest gratitude for writing the book *Your Body's Many Cries for Water.* Since reading your book, I've been drinking water religiously, and have had many positive changes in my body and mind. One of the most important changes is that I am sleeping longer and deeper than before, and the sleep is helping me to heal of course.

Some months after I had breast cancer surgery in 1994, I developed a slight twinge-like sensation in my shoulder. However, since I have been following your advice about drinking water and using salt, the sensation has disappeared. Also, I have an overall sense of better health and well-being.

In retrospect, I remember feeling somewhat weary and sickly, at the same time I was feeling extremely thirsty. I must have been dehydrated most of my 41 years. If I had known how important water was to the workings of every cell, organ and system of the body, then I may not have gotten breast cancer, at least not at this age.

Again I want to thank you for doing such great work, it's strange how the simplest things, i.e. the things right before our eyes, are the ones most difficult to see for most people.
Sincerely, L. L.

Note: As you read, my twenty-two years of research on the pathological outcome of unintentional dehydration of the body exposed a direct and unquestionable relationship between persistent water shortage within the interior of the cells and cancer formation in those cells. In some cases, correcting dehydration and its metabolic complications can reverse the disease process and naturally prevent the recurrence of cancer. You saw it in Drew Bauman's report. My work on this topic is now being recognized. I have on two occasions been asked to address the Cancer Control Society conferences and explain the process. The videotape of my 2002 lecture, *Dehydration and Cancer*, is available, and you can order it on *www.watercure.com*.

Asthma:

I am writing this letter to thank you for sharing your discovery about the need for water with your readers. I have benefited greatly from following your advice on water intake.

The changes in my health have been very noticeable. Asthma used to be a major health concern of mine. Since I have been drinking enough water, however, I have been able to breathe fine without the use of any medication. What a difference this has made in my life. There have been other benefits as well, such as softer skin and increased mental awareness.

I am so happy to have read your book, and I share your advice with as many people as I can. Once again, thank you for your help.
Sincerely, J. W.

Blurred Vision; Skin; Migraine:

In the fall of 1983, I began to have problems with my vision. I went to Dr. Savage in Kingston, PA, and was diagnosed with "floaters." This condition became progressive and I began to become upset. Dr. Savage began looking for different conditions in the body such as Lyme disease and other conditions, but they found nothing and my condition got worse. In January 1994, I went to Wills Eye Clinic, in Philadelphia.

They concluded my problem was caused by ulcerative colitis, which I had about 30 years prior and the new diagnosis was UV-, which is inflammation of the gel of the eyes. My vision was cloudy and blurry; it was like looking through a lace curtain that kept moving, like strings floating in the distance. They prescribed 80 milligrams of Prednisone, a cortisone derivative. They began adjusting doses and I was on Prednisone for two years.

As this went on, I became even more upset. They were telling me the worst cases that could be. They thought maybe it was lymphoma, because it affects the eye immediately. Vision was still cloudy and reading was difficult, I had to wear glasses for reading. Emotionally I was drained and it cost me about $1,000. Every time I had a new appointment, I was a wreck.

Originally the prognosis was that if it didn't clear up, it would get progressively worse and even though I wouldn't go blind, I would have a real problem especially with driving at night. Then, by chance, in December of 1994, I read an article in a newspaper thanking Bob Butts for telling people about Dr. Batman's water cure, that two quarts of water and 1/2-tsp. salt as seasoning on foods and excluding caffeine drinks could cure most diseases. I figured it couldn't hurt to try, it was inflammation, and so I hydrated myself. About two weeks later, after drinking water steadily, I had an appointment with Dr. Savage; he noticed a remarkable difference. I told him about the water cure, but he brushed it off. He concluded the drugs finally worked. I felt it was the water. He told me to stay on the water and come back in a month. Each month got better! By the fourth month, I was completely off the medication that I had been on for two years. My doctor has been keeping an eye on me for the past six months. For the first time in months, I haven't had to have a monthly visit. In addition to that, I just feel so much better! My skin is hydrated, wrinkles diminished and I rarely get the migraine headaches I used to.

As far as I'm concerned, I think water has been a wonderful cure. I tell everyone about the water cure. It certainly can't hurt anyone! And it sure is safer than taking chemicals through soda, coffee and prescriptions. I just drink water.

I know another lady with the same problem and she has improved also. I want to check with her to see how she is progressing. I just talked to her on the phone because she had similar symptom and was upset. She also went to Wills Eye Clinic. She went to the same doctor because she was upset with the doctors here. I told Dr. Jordan in Scranton about my situation; he said it was interesting but that he couldn't believe it was just the water. Whether it was the water and salt completely, I don't know. As of now, I hardly have any wrinkles on my skin. I had tiny wrinkles and they've disappeared. Your whole body and physiological systems change. Everything changes in your body. Now, if I don't drink water, by the third day or fourth day, my vision gets affected again. This makes me believe that it is indeed the water that keeps my vision clear and I see normally. I tell a lot of people about your book *Your Body's Many Cries for Water.*
Sincerely, M. W.

**Cough, Abdominal Pain;
Constipation:**

I have bought and read *Your Body's Many Cries for Water* and wish to write to Dr Batmanghelidj to thank him, as my health has improved from simply drinking ordinary water. It has cured a dry cough that kept me awake at night, tummy pains, and constipation. Today I had to take a urine sample to register at the local NHS (as I have just moved home), and for the first time in my life, my urine was clear. Also, since increasing my salt intake by a pinch each day, there are no more faint spells after a hot bath. I wish to thank him for sharing this profound knowledge with us and am also sharing the information with my family, friends and colleagues and wish him only the best as he helps heal our planet.

Please would you forward this email on to the department at Tagman who liaise with authors.

Thanks in advance, W. T.

Back Pain; Bronchial Constriction; Hypertension.

Thank you for writing the book *Your Body's Many Cries for Water.* By following the principles in it, I have handled my health problems.

Here is a list of my former body somatic:

- Lower back pain
- Neck pain
- Bronchial constriction
- Non-working I/C valve
- Knee pain
- Hypertension

Water and salt completely handled these discomforts!!

To really understand the scope of your book, I had to read it twice. I'm glad I did! Originally I got the book from the Ken Roberts Company and have been disseminating it and the video to my family and friends. People really want this knowledge.

The barriers to getting this principle into general use seem staggering, yet like water on the rock, may it prevail.

You are a leader in the health profession and I salute you.
Best regards, T. E.

♦   ♦   ♦

Angina; Heartburn; Gout:

This letter is in response to the last paragraph on page 164 of your wonderful book *Your Body's Many Cries for Water* in which you asked that if the information in your book has helped, to please write you a note telling how increased water intake has affected people.

Let me begin by stating I first learned of you while listening to the radio program *Coast-to-Coast* AM with Barbara Simpson. She was talking with you and also Bob Butts. At the time, the discussion was about asthma, which affects my grandson, and I proceeded to order your *ABC of Asthma, Allergies, and Lupus* book. After reading only Chapter 1, I immediately ordered more books for family members and friends, and a tape of the radio program. I realized that many of the health disorders I personally endured might be due to dehydration rather than old age (71), so I became a proponent of your new paradigm, began your water and salt cure and within a week I began to see astonishing results.

I no longer suffer from dermatitis, dry patchy skin, dependent edema, so-called fungal infection under my toenails, gout, angina, heartburn (I thought I had hiatal hernia problems until they went away) and dyspepsia! I have lost 5 pounds without dieting and I feel better mentally and physically, presumably because of better metabolism.

My wife suffered for years from swollen lower extremities and the problem has never been diagnosed. After only a few days of your water cure, the swelling disappeared, and she is able to eat ham again!

So please accept my profound gratitude of sharing your discovery with the world.
Very truly yours, R. G.

Heartburn:

Just a brief message to let you know that after just 7 days on 2 liters of water per day plus a half teaspoonful of salt I have experienced a dramatic improvement in my stomach problems—peptic ulcer, heartburn and reflux. I do not have heartburn any more. I think my asthma has also improved. I will provide a more detailed report in about four weeks. Thank you so much for sharing your wonderful health discoveries with me and the rest of the world.
Thank you, L. L.

Note: I received the following two letters from A.C. and included them both because I want to explain the relationship of PMDD to water-metabolism disruption.

Premenstrual Disorders;
Suicidal:

My husband and I are avid health-lovers, and members of the Grain and Salt Society.

Almost 3 years ago I was diagnosed with severe PMDD (Premenstrual Dysphoric Disorder) and clinical depression. I tried *all* the recommended treatments, from Prozac to wonder creams, to herbal concoctions, you name it, and I tried it. *None* of it worked. After 2 and half years of intense suffering, my husband and I discovered Dr F. Batmanghelidj, M.D. and his amazing 'water cure.' After reading his book *Your Body's Many Cries for Water*, the solution to my problems became as clear as day to my husband and me. I started self-medicating with water hydration; Natural Ocean harvested salt from The Grain & Salt Society, pure-grade L-Tryptophan, exercise and nutritional support. It has been 6 months since I started this regimen, and I can say with utter confidence that *all my symptoms have completely disappeared.* For your information, I suffered the following symptoms before this treatment:

- Severe PMS (moodiness, irritability, uncontrolled anger)
- Clinical depression
- Chronic fatigue
- Bloating
- Irregular menstruation
- Hormonal imbalances (testing showed higher than normal prolactin levels, indicating possible prolactin-secreting adenoma)
- Menstrual migraine
- Cravings
- Seasonal allergies

Because of the immense success I had in treating my disorders with these simple natural methods, I have created a web site dedicated to women who suffer from PMDD, and I promote this natural, simple and effective cure heavily. I have also supplied links on my Index page for interested persons to The Grain & Salt Society, and Dr. B's site www.watercure.com.

It is my intention to share this information with as many people as I can, as PMDD is an extremely debilitating condition, with many more women suffering from its effects than is generally known. If Dr B. and Global Health Solutions deem it appropriate, I would appreciate it greatly if they would have a look at my non-profit site and its contents, and help me to promote this natural cure.

In fact, I would be very curious to hear Dr B.'s professional comments about my story of self-healing using his research. My opinion is that conventional medicine is not doing enough to help women with this disorder, and many are led astray by large pharmaceutical corporations' sponsorships of misleading propaganda and promotion of drugs such as SSRIs, without fully researching or making public the real causes and proper treatments for this female malady. I look forward to your comments,
Sincerely, A.C.

I am delighted to hear from you, thank you very much for replying. Yes of course you may use my letter in your new book, this is wonderful! Out of curiosity, what is the title if you don't mind me asking? I would love to read it when it is published. Right now my husband is reading your book *ABC of Asthma, Allergies, and Lupus,* and I am patiently waiting my turn.

As for getting tryptophan without a prescription, this is a long story. My husband and I searched high and low for pure-grade tryptophan; as you know it is so very difficult a product to get hold of without a prescription, but it is not impossible. We knew that we could get it through a doctor's prescription, but being new to the city we live in, we had not yet developed a sufficient relationship with a doctor for me to feel comfortable discussing this unconventional treatment method for my problems. You might understand I had had so many dissatisfying experiences over the past 3 years in this particular arena of my health dealing with conventional medicine that I wanted to circumvent the good doctors where possible. Perhaps some would consider this unwise, but I did not feel that there were any risks. My dear husband and I had done our homework and felt fairly confident that we were on the right track. Anyway, the upshot of it was that we eventually found a company in California that sells pure-grade pharmaceutical tryptophan, at $xx a bottle. Ouch! ;-) But the benefits far outweigh the cost, and that is more important for us. We investigated the company (just to be sure) and everything checked out, so we went ahead bought the tryptophan without prescription.

If you don't mind reading a small novel, I would like to tell you what happened before I started taking the tryptophan supplement, you might find this interesting.

About 6 months ago, before we had found this company to buy from direct, and shortly after reading your book, I had been experimenting with the 'cure' by getting tryptophan into my system through drinking a glass of warm whole milk before bed each night, and again in the morning, then doing 1 hour's brisk walking to get it through the blood brain barrier (as you explained in your book) and another hour's walk in the afternoon, all the while hydrating with water, etc. My husband and I were mightily impressed with the results just from these simple methods. My depression had lifted considerably and I had some energy again (although not yet cured, my symptoms were beginning to alleviate somewhat). We had gone through such a tough time Doc, we were on the edge of divorce many times, we really could not believe that the answer to my health problems could be so simple, so we were proceeding cautiously, thinking this is too good to be true. I continued with the warm milk for about one month, but before long the mucus-forming properties of the milk started aggravating my allergies and I had to stop the warm milk routine. For the next month or so I did fairly well by simply eating the foods that contain tryptophan naturally, but I was by no means as well as I felt I could be if I could get my hands on pure pharmaceutical-grade L-Tryptophan. And as I expected, the real results of this treatment method started showing once I started taking the tryptophan in supplement form (starting with 1000 mg for 2 weeks, then 500 mg, then intermittently and so on).

It feels wonderful to be me again Dr. B. My husband and I refer to you as 'Dr Batman' when we discuss your books and your work, and as this is a term of endearment for us as we have great respect for what you represent. I want to personally say a great big thank you to you dear Dr Batman! Your research and knowledge not only literally helped to save my life (I was *suicidal* at one point, when my PMDD and depression was at its worst), but it was also instrumental in great part to saving a beautiful marriage, my mental health, and not the least, the psychological health of a beautiful 6-year-old boy, who no longer has to be confused and hurt by his Mommy's unexplainable mood swings. Right now I am working through some psychological issues relating to my childhood, which, in my opinion, and according to some of the research I've done, plays a big role in triggering PMDD in some susceptible women. I am moving forward on solid ground at last, instead of treading water always fearing that I would drown from exhaustion (metaphorically speaking).

Dr Batman, what is your professional opinion about Premenstrual Dysphoric Disorder? I think I am on the right track when I say that primarily this disorder is triggered by 'stress,' whether this is life stress or stress through chronic dehydration. Conventional medicine says that PMDD is caused in some women who have an abnormal response to normal hormonal changes. In my humble layman's opinion, I think this is inaccurate, misleading, and nothing more than simple 'shooting into the wind' with nothing more than a theory. Do you know anything about PMDD? Is there a possibility you might do some research about this disorder and publish your findings? It would help so many women and their families, Doc.

I don't think I am that wrong in saying that severe PMS and PMDD has been the cause of many a divorce and other family dysfunction. After all, I have experienced this aspect firsthand. And being a man, you are surely familiar with the jokes about PMS and the stigmatization in our society of this female condition? ☺ PMDD is a very serious condition in my opinion, even life threatening because of the very real possibility of suicide and manslaughter when it reaches its worst levels. Anyone who spends some time speaking to women with PMDD (and their spouses and children) will soon realize the far-reaching effects of PMDD, not only for the sufferer but also for her loved ones as well. The longer PMDD remains untreated (and conventional methods in my opinion are not adequate treatment), the worse it gets, even leading to more serious depressive illnesses. In my opinion people (and the med-ical community) are not taking it seriously enough. I think you can tell I feel quite strongly about this. ;-)

But now I think I have taken up too much of your precious time with my ramblings. ☺

Thank you again Dr. Batman, you are doing humanity a great service with your work. May you always find great happiness and success in all your endeavors.
Sincerely, A. C.

Note: The physiological preparation for the monthly menstrual cycle demands increased water intake and dilution of blood by at least 15 to 25 percent. The blood must be dilute and thin in consistency to pre-vent circulatory disturbance when part of it is shed with the outer layer of endometrium of the uterus. This process involves the water-regula-tory actions of histamine and its subordinate operators. These chemicals not only produce pain but could also influence neuropsycho-logical/physiological activity of the brain. In a book by Carl Pfeiffer called *Nutrition and Mental Health: An Orthomolecular Approach to Balancing Body Chemistry*, histamine has been shown to influence emo-tional states of the body. Additional proof is in the fact that all tricyclic antidepressant drugs are very, very strong antihistamines. However, water and salt are infinitely more effective, natural, and less harmful antihistamines and alleviate the health problems associated with excess histamine activity in the body—hence A. C.'s observations.

🜄 🜄 🜄

Pain; Swelling of Legs:

About eight months ago, I had a talk with Bob Butts, owner of Cee-Kay Auto in Moosic, PA. When Bob discussed the "water cure" with me I laughed, I really laughed. I had this leg problem, where my legs used to swell up really bad; I could hardly walk because of my arthritis and gout. I went to the doctor, and was given anti-inflammatory pills. They just ended up ripping my gut out, so I stopped taking them. Then when Bob talked to me again about your program, I decided to give it a try and start it. I have kept it going for the last six months, and now, I feel like a young person. I am 54 but feels like 20.

My attitude changed greatly after I started drinking water. When you're living in constant pain, your mind is only on one thing. I was just going to get rid of my business and say I can't do what I used to. I usually work 10 to 15 hours a day. I felt I might as well get out of the business. Then I started just drinking water and adding a little salt on my food. My health has really improved in the last four to six months. I am not saying that is all because of the water. Maybe it is, maybe it isn't. All I know is that since I have been following the "water cure" and have made it a habit. I really feel much better and my wife will also tell you that. I used to be nasty and very unpleasant to live with and now all that has changed. Instead of drinking coffee in the morning or milk like I used to, I go home for breakfast and I have a 12-oz glass of water. I don't drink Coke or beer with my meals or anything else except for a 12-oz glass of water. If I want a beer later, then I'll have one.

It is funny, people with swollen legs are told not to drink so much fluid and to stay away from salt, but I did the opposite and my legs are just about down to normal. I can wear cowboy boots again, I haven't worn a pair since I was 44 years old, and that's when my gout got real bad. It was pill after pill until I ended up with ulcers from them and now I don't take any pills.

My joint pain is just about gone. It'll flare up now and again. It's the kind of work that I do. It depends on the stress, especially in the shoulders. I do a lot of heavy work, a lot of pulling; picking up heavy tires and parts all day. Some days you go home and your shoulders hurt, but that's from normal wear and tear.

Before I started on the "water cure" on a scale from one to ten, I felt like checking in, a zero. I wanted to die but now at least I am a seven or eight. Working on getting to a ten; when I get there, I'll let you know. Thank you, M. G.

Bleeding Tongue:

Your book, *Your Body's Many Cries for Water* was mentioned to me several years ago by a co-worker, but I skeptically disregarded this recommendation, having suffered my entire life with a medically unrecognized problem. I was thoroughly disillusioned with all medical professionals. The problem I call "extreme dry mouth" with muscular/tissue hypertension, because I've never seen, heard of or read about a similar case in my 54 years. I now recognize it as a symptom of dehydration.

My tongue first manifested white patches of seemingly dead skin about 17 months of age. Until about 6 weeks ago, other signs of dehydration were obvious (but unrecognizable until I read your book)—constant runny nose, watery eyes, puffed eyelids, susceptible to colds and flu. These latter signs cleared almost immediately once I increased my water intake. By the time I was in school, my entire tongue was coated with a white layer that could be peeled off my tongue in strips often accompanied by skin (membrane), laying bare a raw, sometimes bleeding tongue. No one suggested water—iodine perhaps or yeast medication, but never water. Wisely, I would not allow doctors to experiment with different drug remedies for something they couldn't identify. Aside from my apparent weakened immune system, I was healthy, so just accepted the condition as my lot in life and stopped searching for answers.

I followed the eating principles of Natural Hygiene as outlined in the book by Harvey and Marilyn Diamond *Fit for Life and Living Healthy*. Great emphasis was placed upon eating high-water-content foods and omitting meat, dairy products and concentrated foods from the diet. However, personal circumstances made it impossible for me to adhere to this regimen, and signs of dehydration re-appeared again. Within the past year my tongue has appeared reptilian, skinny, long, hard, shiny and thick at the apex. Living with this diseased state has proven painful and embarrassing, especially the speech distortion caused by the swollen tip (apex) and drooling caused by excessive saliva secretion.

Since June 2001, I have been enjoying eight 10-ounce glasses of water with sea salt each day and although the pain and drooling have gone, my tongue is still swollen in places in spite of daily local massage to increase circulation. The white membrane/dead skin apparently now is developing a healthy pink membranous layer underneath.

Dr. Batmanghelidj, thank you for your intelligent diligence in revealing that chronic dehydration is a causative agent in the production of disease conditions; you have shown great courage and perseverance in dealing with bureaucratic medical "authorities." I thank and admire you greatly.
Sincerely, R. E. N.
Ottawa, Canada

Chest Pain; Constipation:

I just wanted to tell you that your wonderful report on water was a blessing to me. I had been to doctors and no one found anything wrong with me. The results of these tests were 100% great health, but I was so miserable. I had (6 months ago) chest pains and could not go to the bathroom without a laxative. I had accepted the fact that I was to be totally miserable the rest of my life or until something showed up to help me, and that's when your letter arrived. Thank you so very much!!

I started drinking lots and lots of water from the time I read your report. It shocked my socks off, and I could tell the difference by the next day. My exhausted feeling left me and I was even getting up in the middle of the night. I never got up at night to go to the bathroom before, but still felt exhausted. Now I get up in the night, yet I feel awake and alert the next day. Your reports are terrifically done. One week on the water program (6–8 glasses) I had my first bowel movement without the aid of a laxative and have continued so. I had never in my 43 years dreamt I'd be excited about a bowel movement, but I am in heaven about this wonderful change to my system. I wanted to be sure and write and thank you for your fantastic reports. You are saving people and that is a special gift.

Keep up the good work!!!
Sincerely yours, G. P. A.

Constipation:

After reading your book a couple of weeks ago, I have tried to drink a glass (one cup, 8 oz) of water per waking hour.

I am 68 years old and for months have just generally felt bad. I'd go to bed at night feeling creaky. After a fitful sleep, I'd wake up the next morning feeling like I had been run over by a truck. Throughout the day, my energy would flag and everything I did seem to take a concerted effort.

About 17 months ago I had a cancerous kidney removed along with a bothersome gall bladder. Checkups reveal no more cancer. I just thought my aches and pains and lack of energy were a result of my age and the stress of the surgeries.

Not so! After about four days on the water cure, I began to experience a general feeling of well-being and began to have energy throughout the day and to sleep well at night. After two weeks, I feel like a fully functioning human being again!

My thanks to you and your book for getting me back on this logical, commonsense routine of drinking plenty of water.

By the way I found your book *Your Body's Many Cries for Water* through Dr. Lorraine Day's website (www.drday.com).
Sincerely yours, G. L. S.

      💧   💧   💧

Night Sweat; Hot Flashes:

I had the book *Your Body's Many Cries for Water* recommended to me and seriously increased my water intake. The benefit I am finding is that my hot flashes and night sweats have dropped dramatically. I am 55 years of age, post-menopausal and was having considerable trouble with both, 24 hours a day. The night sweats have improved so much that I am now sleeping much better; another plus, not waking many times each night. As soon as I feel a hot flash starting I drink a small amount of water and it subsides. With so many women on HRT these days it would be good if this message could be included on your web site. If you want any more information from me you can contact me on my email. Regards, M.

Dry Eyes:

I am amazed and grateful for your materials. After years of eye discomfort, I went to my optometrist for the lachrymal occlusion procedure. He ran a test of the water content around my eyes and said on a scale of 1 to 20, with 10 being symptomatic of "dry-eye syndrome," I was a 4. He diagnosed me with Sjogren's syndrome. He put temporary plugs in the tear ducts of one eye—these would dissolve in five days and, in a subsequent appointment, I would report if I felt relief before the permanent plugs were put in.

I read up on Sjogren's and found I had other symptoms. About two days into the test, I saw a brochure about your theories. I immediately began drinking water as suggested; my prior routine might include three glasses a day, sodas, and coffee. At my return appointment, three weeks later, I asked for another test before the plugs were implanted—one eye was an 8 and one was a 10! He said it was not appropriate for him to proceed and asked what I was doing. I gave him your book. He has asked to retest me in 90 days. He said "dry-eye syndrome" causes many patients lots of discomfort and problems. I hope he will pass my experience on to other patients. I am anxious for the retest to validate my experience empirically.

I also feel better than I have in years. I had frequent nosebleeds, which have stopped. I don't crave caffeine and I have no constipation. I have lost weight, and I am certain I am just beginning to reap the benefits of your program. I have bought several books for friends with asthma and hypertension. It all makes such good sense.
Thank you so much, L. A.

Sight:

As I told you about a month ago my boyfriend Bob lost his sight because he has M.S., well, he has gained his sight back (20/40) by using your suggestions of water, carrot juice, vitamin E and B.

The doctor at the N.E. Eye Institute could not believe that Bob's eyesight came back.
Thank you for your help. K. S.

      ♦   ♦   ♦

Salt:

How do I start? How do I begin to thank you for saving my mother's life? Had we not spoken on the phone and had you not expanded on the data in your book, I firmly believe my mother would be dead. With the salt/water data and our frequent discussions, I believe you have given her a second chance to rehabilitate and recuperate.

When her sodium was 108 (140 is normal) your directions brought her up to 127, in effect rescuing her from the edge of death. When she had pneumonia, your insight saved her life. When her doctor said she had only two options—using so little water that her kidneys would fail or using more water and dropping her sodium back to a dangerous level, you came up with the third option, using an onion extract to help her kidneys retain sodium. With that knowledge I have been able to keep her sodium level at 130 and increase her water to about 2900 cc's a day. Even with the medication she was on and the 40 mg Lasix twice a day, the salt and water have had a significant effect on her health and her edema.

It has also helped me tremendously with the amount of stress that I am under every day. Thank you Dr. Batmanghelidj—from both of us from the bottom of our hearts.
Sincerely, John & Mom

Opinion:

Thank you for your gifts! Your gift of knowledge is the best of all. Patients are now coming back for office visits after I have told them about water. They are getting better. I believed you, but it nice to get confirmation from patients.

To date, I have not been given the courtesy of a reply from Joel D. Wallach, B.S., D.V.M., and M.D. There does not appear to be any scientific evidence for his claims. Hopefully I am wrong about this. Your name has been used in conjunction with Dr. Wallach's; you may want to be careful, since there is so much controversy with his outlandish claims. Your reputation is good, and best kept that way.

In general, I am very open-minded, but I do not anticipate that any scientific evidence will arise to change my opinion.

Anyway, keep up the great work the Lord has given you. My work involves chronic Lyme disease, intestinal yeast, low metabolism bioelectric medicine, and others. Your work is making mine easier.
Thanks, Charles L. Crist, M.D.

Migraine; Eyes:

Thank you, thank you, and thank you! Thank you for discovering the simplest and greatest miracle cure ever. And thank you for all your years of hard work—no words are adequate. The migraines that destroyed my life for 35 years, and my pocketbook are gone-gone-gone-gone (One of which I would never have dreamed about).

I've been wearing glasses practically all my life (now bifocals) and every year I need stronger glasses—when suddenly two weeks ago my glasses felt awkward somehow—again believing I needed a stronger prescription, I went for a check-up. To my shock both eyes got better (upper and lower) and for the first time in my life my glasses are weaker and my eyes stronger.

There have been many other unexpected changes—feel better all over, look better, sleep better, think better, etc. etc. How dehydrated I must have been is unreal—and how dehydrated most everyone is, is truly tragic. I can SEE it in almost all the people I know and meet. Therefore, I talk about WATER constantly and I speak of Dr. Batmanghelidj all the time and my prayer is that the two will soon be known throughout the world, for it is truly God's greatest miracle cure.

Thank you dear Dr. Batmanghelidj—thank you for my life.
Sincerely, M. A. V.

◊   ◊   ◊

Restless Legs; Salt:

I have just finished reading your book *Your Body's Many Cries for Water.* All that I can say is THANK YOU!! I have suffered with restless legs for 15–20 years, I wake up in the middle of the night and I have to exercise my legs. I have gone to my regular M.D. and to my neurologist and neither could help me. They have prescribed different exercises for me to do but these didn't seem to do the trick. I have tried a TENS unit and many over-the-counter medications & quinine water. Nothing helped!! Then my son gave me your book and I read with great interest p. 157 on Ease of Sleeping. Now I drink 8–10 glasses of water each day, and before I go to bed I put a pinch of salt on my tongue. I had decreased my salt intake next to nothing because my husband's doctor had recommended that he go on a low-salt diet, I also went along with him. Since reading your book we both have upped our salt intake now; I have nervous legs once, maybe twice, a month where it used to happen two to three times a night. I am so glad that I read your book and I have told many others about it and my wonderful results.
Sincerely, R. B.

Opinion:

Surely you will be nominated for a Nobel Prize, but in what category? It could not be medicine, for we don't want water and salt to be declared to be medicinal drugs!! The FDA and AMA would want to have them dispensed "by prescription only."

Since about 1930 American drugs, artificial foods and environmental chemicals (when added to the dumb-down educational system) have changed self-reliant, responsible, clear-thinking citizens into sick and sore zombies. Thank you for choosing this needy country for your grass roots health-information campaign.

Perhaps you will be awarded the Nobel Peace Prize for ending all wars, when everyone gets sufficiently hydrated to be mentally stable, pain-free and content.
Yours truly, J. R.

Opinion:

Your Body's Many Cries for Water is by far the best I have read in my 75 years. My experience with the new diseases such as carpal tunnel syndrome, electro-sensitivity and childhood leukemia has shown a more-than-coincidental relationship to low water consumption and EMF exposure.

The enclosed copy of research by a Swedish scientist postulates how EMF damages cells, my experience shows that those with high water consumption are less susceptible to this damage. Cells banging into each other 60 times a second could be squeezing the water out.

I have always been a large water drinker and at 75 have been healthy, energetic and not hospitalized since appendicitis at age 15, and my wife has always avoided drinking water, been lethargic, five artery bypasses, heart attack, arthritis etc. Since following the instructions in your book, I notice an improvement in her energy level, cognition and spirit in just a few weeks.

Should you be interested I have much research data and a bibliography of source material that I would be pleased to send you.

Your reaction to these suppositions would be appreciated. Again, congratulations on a tremendous book.
Sincerely yours, J. A. F.

♦ ♦ ♦

Chronic Fatigue:

First of all I would like to thank you very much for the information contained in your book *Your Body's Many Cries for Water,* which my husband received a short while back.

I have suffered from M.E. (in America, chronic fatigue) for the last seven years. By following a variety of alternative treatments I have managed to survive all these years in spite of my limitations. Since increasing the amount of water I drink as you suggest (only four weeks now), I have experienced a very marked improvement in my energy levels as well as having less pain or perhaps no more pains!! It is still early stages, but I am delighted with the results and I thought you would be pleased to know of this.

I have told many of my friends and neighbors about your book. On the other hand I would like to order a copy of your book to be sent directly to a very good friend who just came out of the hospital, due to a heart condition.

I thank you again for your help.
Gratefully yours, M. F.

Allergies; Dry Skin:

My fluid intake was fine, but it was NOT water, and I have learned that WATER IS THE KEY. Besides my heartburn and allergy problems that have been virtually eliminated, I have noticed other things as well. For instance, just the other morning I realized that it would be around this time of year that I would find my skin so absolutely dry that it would hurt. I would notice this mostly on my forehead as well as on the backs of my hands. I would then borrow some of my wife's facial/hand lotion to restore the moisture and that would even hurt when I applied it because my skin was so extremely dry.

Like I say, it was just the other morning that I realized that I didn't have this problem this winter. Also, my contact lens comfort has improved considerably. I notice this mostly after having worn them for a long period of time. I no longer get that "my eyes are tired and I got to get these lenses out," type feeling. My complexion is much better too (less pimples/blackheads). Hard bowel movements are a thing of the past now, and oh yes, my knees, I just thought it was part of getting old, if I sat with my legs crossed or sat with my legs folded under me for even a short time, when I get up, my knees would really hurt as I straightened my legs out. It was like a s-l-o-w straightening out was all I could muster. Like I say, I assumed it was part of getting old. Well last month I realized that the flexibility in my knees has been restored. They flex so easily now.

The adage about getting better as opposed to getting older, applies to me! Water has made such a positive change in my life that I believe it may apply to anyone who may not be taking in enough water.

It has been wonderful to feel these changes, which is why I am quite happy to share what I have learned from Dr. Batmanghelidj. I'll be sure to let you know if my doctors say anything about my letter and Dr. Batman's book that I gave them.
Sincerely, T. L.

Prostate Cancer:

I am writing to thank you for leading me through the cure of prostate cancer.

During a flight physical in July 1999 my PSA was at 4.6. I was referred to an urologist that led to a biopsy, which came back positive in October. I went to Walter Reed Medical Center for a second opinion in January 2000 where my PSA was found to be at 5.7 and it was confirmed as cancer.

While home for Christmas, my mother kept talking about your book, *Your Body's Many Cries for Water.* I finally asked her to please stop talking about it so I could enjoy the holidays and my granddaughters, but I promised to read the material she gave me on the flight back to Germany. While I was at Walter Reed in Washington, D.C., I found out all I could about possible cures and facilities or clinics that might serve as alternative resources, because everyone I talked to wanted to operate. Actually, three choices were recommended to me: wait and watch, radiation therapy, and surgery, which was their strongest recommendation.

I began drinking water while at Walter Reed as a result of downloading your volumes of information from the Internet at *www.watercure.com.* I e-mailed you because I had some questions, and when I returned to Europe I found an answer from you inviting me to call you at your office, which I did. You asked me many questions and told me to begin drinking water, carrot juice, orange juice, use salt (which I had not done for twenty years), eat lots of vegetables and fruits and the only eating restriction you gave me was to not eat fried foods. You also told me to give up coffee, alcohol and sodas. You told me to walk for an hour in the morning and an hour at night, faithfully. You invited me to call you whenever I had questions and when I asked what it would cost, you stated there would be no charge . . . . . WOW!!!

Since then I have called regularly, every week at first and about once a month more recently. I have had monthly PSA tests run and they generally have been within safe tolerance since February (the first month after beginning the water cure). In March I went to Panama and Vietnam and was not able to follow the regime faithfully but I did keep drinking my daily amount of water and my PSA was slightly elevated when it was tested in April. I went back to the regime and the PSA was way down the next month.

I went to Panama for a family reunion in late July and early August, where I drank some beer and coffee and when I returned to Europe I found my PSA was up again. This concerned me and I called to speak with you about it. In our conversation you questioned me very closely about the consumption of alcohol and I confessed that since I live in Germany where the world's best beers are available, I usually had one or two at dinner. You told me not to drink any alcohol and I obeyed. You also shared with me that the high PSA indicated a higher acidity in my body and recommended that I eat lots of vegetables, particularly green ones, to cause a higher PH. The next month's test was at 3.3.

At first when I attempted to explain what I am doing to medical doctors they basically blew me off, but more recently I have spoken to a few who are interested. Since beginning this suggested regime, I have really felt better than before I started. I was in pretty good shape, but within three weeks, I noticed that when I did the same cardiovascular exercises as before, I had to work much harder to raise my heart beat to the normal 150 that I had always achieved before. It would only reach 130 with the same effort. I asked you about this and you told me it was because my heart muscles were probably dehydrated before and no longer have to work so hard. With the same effort now, I only achieve a heart rate of 115 to 120.

For years I have had some pains in my knees and in one hip when I walked or ran and my knees hurt when I walked after getting up out of a chair . . . . This was completely gone after about three months of water drinking. My nagging lower back pain has disappeared and I really feel great. I am 60 and quite frankly I feel about as good as I did at 40 and I am cured of prostate cancer.

I was raised on a farm, flew fighters, built houses and commercial buildings and owned a number of construction consulting businesses in my adult years, so from my experience I am a practical thinker and water makes sense. I can personally claim that your information works and it is amazing that so many other friends of mine think it is just too simple a solution. It is particularly distressing to encounter the ignorance shown by traditional medical people who seem to be blinded by their training and professional arrogance when it comes to acceptance of your information. Thank you very much Dr. Batmanghelidj and I pray that "WE" are successful in getting your practical information heard by people who can benefit from it.

Please feel free to share this information with anyone it will benefit.
Respectfully, W. J.

Cancer of the Tonsil:

First I want to thank you profusely for writing that book! I can relate to your struggles with the medical establishment as I have opted for alternative methods other than chemo, radiation & surgery and have had to endure what I call the Western medical gauntlet, which is yet another story.

I don't know you, but I'm proud of you! You're one of the real heroes!

Some background: In April of 1997 I was diagnosed with squamous cell carcinoma of the left tonsil, which metastasized into the lymph nodes of the neck by Stanford tumor board. I was told I was in the most dramatic way, that I had a 15 to 30% chance of survival if I followed their recommendations. These were to have a radical neck dissection, which included removing the 11th cranial nerve, part of the jaw, and a lot of tissue in my throat, then radiation and 16 weeks of chemo. If I failed to follow recommended procedures my life span was expected to be over within a short 5 weeks! No one would give me a straight answer on costs, but it was reluctantly and unofficially estimated at $350,000 BEFORE the chemo. (By the way, I had an excellent health policy, which almost became my death sentence.)

After thoroughly looking at the options, I bailed out on the surgery, chemo and the radiation. I started an organic macrobiotic diet, got rid of the toxins in and around my house, cleaned up my lifestyle, used some herbs, chi-gong and eventually hyperbaric oxygen, which was very effective.

In the last 4 & a half years, I had the cancer looking like it was in remis-sion, but then after a couple of years I slowly fell off the diet. The cancer started up again with four new tumors. I stopped it on this sec-ond occasion with the same regimen for many months, but could not reverse it. A doctor convinced me to cut back on the salt and in a few months I developed 6 more tumors. Up until now, I've never had much pain, or have ever lost a day of work. 20 days ago it has taken a jump-start. Tumors have definitely grown. They may be encroaching on the carotid artery and probably the main nerve sheath. Some necrotizing tissue appeared on the tonsil, covering it within 3 days, possibly some bone loss in the jaw, and the worst part of it, some excruciating stab-bing nerve pain that's off the scale. My latest prognosis was that within days I'd be sucked into the system with overwhelming pain or that I would bleed to death any time.

I just read your 1992 edition of *Your Body's Many Cries for Water* and got a strong feeling this cancer is due to long-term dehydration. I have drunk very little water in the past. I was given OxyContin for pain as well as Percocet. I don't like feeling the drug stupor so I opted to try two glasses of water & a pinch of salt as your book suggested. Amazingly, the water is much more effective for this kind of core pain than the drugs! In only 12 days, there is a change coming on in the tumors. They appear to be shrinking slightly, in any case, softening and changing to smoother shapes. The pain is dramatically disappearing.

This may be too early to say, but the necrotizing tissue on the tonsil seems to be clearing up. Thanks to your book, I hope I've discovered this in time, that ordinary water may be the missing link. Won't that be a tes-tament if I can cure this cancer with your water cure??? The race is on.

So far, I've let the pain dictate my water consumption once I've drunk a liter & a half. This has brought me to 3 - 4 liters a day. I am a 52-year-old scuba charter boat captain and in excellent shape, other than this pesky cancer.
Thank you
Respectfully, E. C.

Muscular Dystrophy:

Around November 1st, 1994, my legs were giving out. They became black and blue from my knees to my thighs and very painful. I went to the doctor and he told me that my muscle enzymes were at 660 and normal was 90. Then I went to see another doctor, and he said that I had muscular dystrophy.

I started talking to you, who told me to start drinking 2 quarts of water daily. I have been, I feel much better and all symptoms disappeared within two months. I also use sea salt liberally with all my meals.

I went back to the doctor and had additional blood work done. The enzyme levels in my muscles were back to normal and the doctor couldn't understand how it was possible. As of this date, March 15, 1995, I am free of all discomfort and symptoms. I also have more energy and better health than I can remember for a long time.
Sincerely, E. D.

Note: Up to this date, May 2003, E. D. has been in remission with no recurrence of his original symptoms.

◊   ◊   ◊

Prostate; Sleep;
Fungal Infection:

I recently read your book *Your Body's Many Cries for Water* and I have seriously been following your advice since the first of January, drinking 8–10 glasses of water per day.

Three things have happened to me physically since I started following your advice. First, the prostate problems that I have had for more than eight years seem to be getting much, much better. As you can see I live in a high, dry place. Prior to your book I could not sleep through the night because of the dryness in my nose and mouth. Now, I have no problems. Finally, the fungus that I have had under my toe nails since the Korean War is gone!

I know many more important things have been reported to you, but these were important to me. I appreciate all the work you're doing. Regards, R. D. B.

◊   ◊   ◊

Bone Marrow Cancer:

In November 1988, I was diagnosed with bone marrow cancer and was told that my condition was terminal. For twelve years, I did not receive any type of chemotherapy.

Doctors do not understand how I can live so long with terminal cancer. Most patients with this type of cancer normally live three to six years, which was the life expectancy they gave me. They cannot understand why I do not have holes in my bones by now.

On August 4, 2000, I was taken to Parkway Medical Center's ER in the following condition:

- Unconscious
- Respiratory failure
- Fever, temperature 104.8
- Heartbeat was 222 beats per minute
- Blood pressure 200/130
- Pneumonia
- Bacterial meningitis (inflammation of the spinal cord and the lining of the brain)
- Blood was sludge
- Hemorrhaging from the nose
- Multiple melanomas (bone cancer)
- Zero immune system (due to bone cancer)

That same week it was reported on television that two healthy young men ages 17 and 21 died of meningitis. The doctors said that if I had arrived at the hospital two hours later I would have been dead upon arrival. Bacterial meningitis is the worse kind of meningitis a person can contract.

I was in ICU for ten days, unconscious and on a ventilator. The doctors did not think I was going to live. The primary-care physician informed my family that I might need a tracheotomy, having a feeding tube placed in my intestines, and be kept alive by machines. My family was informed that I might be a vegetable if and when I did wake up. The doctors said that most patients that have been unconscious and on the ventilator for the length of time I was, usually wake up brain dead.

By the grace of God, on the 11th day I woke up breathing on my own with all my facilities and a sound mind. Today, nine weeks later, I stand in God's amazing grace giving Him all the praise and all the glory. I am healed, walking in divine health. I am also still drinking a gallon and half of water with 1-tsp. of salt every day. Thanks to your teaching. Sincerely, M. J.

Prostate Cancer:

You will appreciate that Ken and I were not so much concerned with constructing a clinical record as we were with bringing to Ken's diagnosis of advanced, untreatable prostate cancer every healing resource that we could muster. I've reconstructed the events as best as I can from supplier invoices, Medicare documents, physicians' bills and so forth. I'm also enclosing a photocopy of the lab reports developed from blood drawings and urine samples in Houston, TX.

PSA readings on June 4 and July 9 and the biopsy taken on July 9 certainly confirm Dr. Syperd's recommendations that Ken should forego any kind of treatment and expect to die within 18 months of the prostate cancer. I ordered your books, videotapes and audiotapes on July 6 and likely received them about July 14. I ordered ConcenTrace on July 13 and probably received it about July 21.

No doubt at all exists that Ken's experience with increased water intake began after the second PSA reading (50.8) was taken. In my recollection Ken began the regimen the day after your book and videotapes were received. For five days Ken's urine was such a dark brown and so dankly smelly that we were alarmed. "It's the cancer cells being expelled," I encouraged him. Ken was sweating profusely and with an acrid, repellent odor. He had to change his bed linens and his clothes (after a shower) several times a day. Ken was drinking from 11 to 13 glasses (8 oz water in a 10 oz glass) of home-distilled water each day. He began each day as you suggest with two glasses of water. Abruptly in the mid-afternoon of the fifth day, Ken's urine appeared clear and his sweating diminished and returned to its ordinary odor.

Exactly when Ken began adding ConcenTrace to our home-distilled water I can't be certain. Ken didn't like the taste of 30 drops/gallon and for a few days he experimented with the amount, finally settling on 18 drops/gallon.

Ever since we purchased the home distiller from Sears several years ago I've been nagging him to enhance the water with minerals. In 1967 I had collapsed with clinical depression, which in 1970 was attributed to a gross calcium/magnesium imbalance resulting from my drinking water treated by a Culligan water softener. Since those days, I've been dedicated to mineral supplements. Ken, however, had done nothing to replace the minerals lost by distilling our water.

When the pre-treatment PSA report came back to the Burzynski Clinic in Houston, Ken was asked how his PSA could have dropped so dramatically, Ken brought the question to me, and it was several days before I realized that the only thing different between the 2nd PSA reading and the 3rd was his greatly increased water intake. Ken had always drunk copious amounts of coffee each day, but only one glass of water, and that's with his dinner.

Ken's tumor appears to be defeated, and the cancer cells in his bone tissue appear to be retreating. Ken continues to drink 8 glasses of water each day.

You are welcome to use any of these documents in any way you wish. Sincerely, C. B.

**Depression; Allergies;
Weight Loss; Energy Surge:**

I read your interview with Dr. Batmanghelidj a couple of weeks ago and it made a profound impression on me. I gave up beverages containing caffeine. Although I have only been on this program for a couple of weeks, I feel like a new person!

I wanted to tell you about some results that I got, because the ones that impressed me the most and for which I am most thankful, are not physical results, per se, they are emotional/psychological and I did get some very good physical results; I lost weight, my allergy symptoms disappeared, and I enjoyed a tremendous upsurge in energy—but I was much more grateful for (and amazed by) a release from a lifelong battle with depression and other emotional and psychological problems.

I had gotten to the point where my nerves were just shot. I was nearly sensitive and overreacted to everything. The slightest setback became a major setback. I couldn't cope with the pressures of even ordinary everyday living, much less more stressful situations. I developed a very short fuse, I would get irritated and angry at the slightest provocation, and then I would get depressed and hated myself, and really just wanted to die. I was ruining my closest relationships, and I contemplated suicide many times.

I began to believe that I might have a mental illness. I saw many different psychiatrists and social workers, but my experiences never really changed. I was progressively more volatile with drastic mood swings, and I lived under a big dark cloud. But then, when I began to follow Dr. Batmanghelidj's guidelines, I felt the big dark cloud lift. It was as if the sun finally came out. I felt calmer and more peaceful, more centered and grounded, and just plain happier.

My nerves no longer jumped out of control at every little thing and I began to feel a profound sense of joy and relief. I no longer felt so much like something was drastically wrong with me. I began to be able to hold my head up and face the world, instead of tending toward a sort of paranoid agoraphobia.

I don't know whether other people with similar problems might get the same relief, but as you say, when you've tried everything else and it's failed, it can't hurt to try something like this. I know many people who don't even drink one glass of water in a day. I can't imagine anyone who wouldn't benefit from increasing his or her intake of water.

Thank you so much for publishing that fascinating interview. It made more sense than anything else I have ever read on health (and I've read a lot), and it has helped me more than anything else I have ever tried (and I've tried a lot!).

Also, a glass of water is free—my last psychiatrist was $65.00 for 45 minutes!! Thank you again,
Sincerely yours, K. M.

◊   ◊   ◊

Knee Pain; Arthritis Pain; Depression; Suicidal; Osteoporosis; Angina; Acid Reflux; Salt; Anxiety Attacks; Weight Loss; Asthma:

I am 67 years old, a mother and a housewife. Ever since I reached 40 years old my health had not been good although I was not terribly sick in bed. I had a knee injury and had suffered with arthritis pain for over 30 years. I don't believe in taking medication for controlling pain. For that reason I stayed away from doctor visits as much as possible in my life.

I had been on a low-salt diet for the last 20 years, believing that salt is not good for health. I had suffered with muscle cramps, acid reflux, constant tiredness, shortness of breath, osteoporosis (as measured by a bone density test), angina pain, pain in my legs in walking, migraine headaches, hot flashes, double vision, arthritis, high cholesterol, depression, etc.

In November 2000 I fell into a very bad depression. I could not cope with my everyday life, couldn't eat or sleep and I was very suicidal. Out of desperation I made a visit to see my doctor and began to take antide-pressant medicine. It seemed to help me for a few days, but my condition became worse as time went on. I started to have terrible anx-iety attacks on top of my depression. I was told by my doctor I may have to live with my medication for the rest of my life because of the chemi-cal imbalance problem in my brain.

I didn't believe my doctor's explanation. After three weeks of my trial with antidepressant medicine I completely stopped taking medicine and seeing my doctor all together. I prayed to God for an answer. Three days later, in May 2001, I accidentally saw Dr. Lorraine Day's interview on TV. She was talking about her recovery from breast cancer. Her drinking large amount of water was one of the key factors contributing to her recovery, as she had not been a big water drinker.

It struck me in that moment, because I had not been a big water drinker either, that I might have the same dehydration problem. I always drank fruit juices, tea, milk and fresh fruits, including watermelons to quench my thirst. I drank very little pure water. I immediately got your book and started drinking two quarts of water with ? teaspoon of salt a day. I eliminated all other liquids for thirst. My depression disappeared in two days. My energy level surged. I noticed foods digested better too. Suddenly I felt alive again. All my other symptoms gradually disap-peared over a six-month period. I couldn't believe the change.

My cholesterol level had gone up to 297. By September 2002 it meas-ured 179. It's now been two years and I am free from all pain and I walk three to six miles per day. I also changed my diet and have lost weight during the past year, dropping from 150 to 130 pounds. I am 5' 1" tall, so that is a good weight for me. I am happy, have a very positive and grateful attitude and love to share my experience with everyone about the water cure and the benefits of a healthful diet and exercise. My husband is 5' 9" and also dropped from 180 to 150 pounds, and is the picture of health at the age of 71. Neither of us takes any medications, which is pretty unusual for people of our age.

My grandson, 12 years old, had very bad asthma, allergies and earaches since he was 5 years old. I introduced the water and salt treatment to him two years ago. He is free from all these now. He is a very healthy and happy child today. My granddaughter, 9 years old, is also drinking water with a little salt and was able to prevent her asthma problem at the beginning stages.

I am so thankful for Dr. Batmanghelidj's discovery on the role of water and salt in the body. When I read his book *Your Body's Many Cries for Water*, everything made so much sense to me. I can't say thank you enough. You are truly God's messenger. Thank you again. You may use my letter as you see fit.
Sincerely, M. F.

Heartburn; Depression; Headaches:

I want to write and tell you of my health improvements since following your water treatment. For the last 10 years I have suffered with chronic heartburn. I have been to many doctors, had numerous tests, even had my gall bladder removed and been prescribed several medications with no relief. I also have had a lifelong problem with depression, have tried many types of therapy and mind-altering drugs, and have been hospitalized. I have been seeing a homeopath, Dr. James J. Berryhill, and he has helped me with several situations. He sent me a copy of your article in *The Last Chance Health Report* Vol. 3 #5, and suggested I also purchase your book *Your Body's Many Cries for Water*. He said he felt this would greatly help me. At that time, I had just been in the hospital having more tests and was beginning a program of several strong medications, some of which had dangerous potential side effects.

On August 24, 1993, I began drinking lots of water, 12 glasses on average and noticed dramatic improvement almost immediately. The heartburn was still occurring at the same rate, but I drank water and found it took 7 minutes for the heartburn to abate. I was dubious, to say the least, but decided not to take any medication and see what happened. After a week or so I noticed I had not been depressed either. This to me was amazing, considering all the advice I had been given in psychological counseling. A few days later, I realized I had not been having headaches as I usually did. I would have a slight headache on a daily basis. I've also noticed my skin is a lot clearer, I have more energy and overall I just feel better.

I have spent untold amounts of money, time away from work (I had used all my vacation time being sick) and energy dealing with medical doctors and hospitals, and receiving minimal relief. I am also in a few very stressful situations, but am able to cope. And I am taking no medication for heartburn or anti-depressants. The episodes of heartburn are fewer now as well. The only change I've made is to drink lots of water. I have not yet begun the rest of your regimen, orange juice, etc., but intend to do so.

I feel like a different person, more in control of my life. It's now been two months and my skepticism is no longer there. I believe in your treatment, and want to thank you for it. I am now telling friends and co-workers to at least try it and have had good reports from them also. September 13, 1993 I had a follow-up appointment with my gastroenterologist, I told her I was feeling a lot better and gave her a copy of your article to read, she was nonplussed.

I am and have been very angry with the medical profession. Doctors for the most part do not even ask about your water intake or diet. Their methods ensure you a return appointment with lingering ailments and no education on being able to take care of yourself. Your treatment is simple, inexpensive, and it works! It is also a threat to medical doctors as they will see less of you and make less money. What I have been through is outrageous and insulting to my intelligence.

Thank you so much for enlightening me on how I can feel better without all the frustration, pain and side effects I've experienced.
Sincerely, S. M.

💧   💧   💧

Depression; Numbness and Tingling:

I am writing to you because I recently purchased a copy of your book, *Your Body's Many Cries for Water*, which without a doubt is one of the best books I have ever read. I feel that your dedication set the tone for the whole book. The information therein has helped me personally, it has assisted me in a report on food additives I have just completed for a magazine, and I am confident that it will help me at some stage when I resume my holistic health practice, which is on hold whilst I finish bringing up my children on my own.

About six years ago, I had two traumatic experiences within two months of each other, following which I suffered a number of symptoms, including numbness and tingling in my arms and hands each morning, recurrent depression, and a craving for carbohydrates and sweet things. I was able to control these somewhat by taking great care about my diet. After reading your book, I decided to drink at least three liters of water a day, keeping a bottle on the floor by my desk and by my bedside at night. Since doing so, I have had a dramatic improvement in my symptoms. My depression has been less frequent and less able to take a hold, the symptoms in my arms are less severe, my energy has been up consistently, and I have been better able to keep up my motivation regarding my diet. My problems have never included weight gain, but my body has sometimes been rather flabby and low in muscle tone. I have noticed that if on a particular day I forget to drink the required amount of water, my symptoms recur or the improvement is less marked. I am trying therefore to keep up the habit.

I found your remarks about aspartame very helpful in writing my report. I understand that this and food additives are very hazardous and that their approval rests on studies which have been widely criticized. Indeed, aspartame and monosodium glutamate, from what I have read, do appear to be implicated in many neurological and behavioral symptoms, and I wonder if train drivers and footballers could be among the people affected by them. I always avoid them, having suffered a very nasty attack after a chop-suey meal in 1976.

I particularly appreciated your book because the therapy does not suppress the human being's power to heal. You are most welcome to use my name and comments as a testimonial of the water therapy.
Yours sincerely,
D. R. H., BA, CertED, LCH

Migraine; Depression; Asthma;
Joint Pain; Chronic Fatigue; Sinusitis;
Gluten Intolerance:

I just found your book *Your Body's Many Cries for Water.* It made a big impression on me—like getting hit between the eyes and now I see!!

I am 39 and have been chasing symptoms of dehydration most of my life—migraines, joint/growing pains, sinusitis, mild asthma, recurrent pneumonia, chronic tiredness, depression, mysterious allergies (recently diagnosed with gluten intolerance), low thyroid. I was treated as a hypochondriac by doctors, given Valium as a kid, told I had to live with my sinusitis, told not to eat wheat, lived with migraines after all treatments failed, criticized by family for not "snapping out of my depression and lethargy." Yet something inside me has kept me looking for the mysterious reason for all these symptoms, which I believed were not normal and which I believed were indicators of distress and therefore not to be "ignored and lived with." You have given me the missing puzzle piece.

I have been struggling to keep my sinuses manageably clear (infection free) by severely limiting gluten in my diet. After 2 days of increased water and salt, my sinuses were 100% clear (wonderful feeling), my breathing was easier (I did not realize how chronically reduced it was) and I have much more energy generally, and my mind is clearer too. Six days and I feel great. Here is the punch line for me—I have been eating wheat these past days. Therefore my gluten intolerance seems to have disappeared with increased water and salt! I am so amazed and excited that I wrote to my naturopath and told her of your book and my experience—she has many patients with the same diagnosis.

My children and my husband are benefiting from more water and salt. In particular my youngest son (6 years old) is much better. I have been chasing the cause of his chronic tiredness, anemia, sinusitis, pneumonia, and ear infection for his whole life. His doctor kept telling me "he is just a sick kid, so accept that and move on."

My husband has chronic high blood pressure and had recently been put on a diuretic, which failed to reduce the pressure, so his doctor doubled the dose, without success. He has also been trying to lose weight with "diet products." He is now on water and salt and his complexion is much better, the whites of his eyes are less bloodshot. No more diet sodas either.

It has only been 6 days so we have a long path ahead, but I am amazed at what I have seen in my family and myself already. I was beginning to think I would acquire some dreadful label like lupus or chronic fatigue syndrome, but instead I have finally found the path to health. It is strange how the Almighty works—I had been praying for guidance to the path to health and went to the bookstore to find a book on lupus, but could not find a decent book, so was walking out when your book caught my eye.

I am so excited by the huge impact and consequences of your information that I am telling my friends and family.

I am a licensed massage therapist; so get to see clients for various relaxation and medical reasons. Your information is going to make a big appearance in my work. I was especially interested in your chapter on stress and dehydration. Since de-stressing folks is a lot of my business, it is natural for me to direct them to your information. I have contacted the school I trained at because I think we could have really benefited from your information in our training. I am urging the school, to at a minimum, include your book on their recommended reading list.

My sister is a physical therapist in South Africa—I directed her to your information too. She tells of many South Africans finding they have better energy when they take salt pills, but that, because of the current trend to reduce sodium, the salt pills are difficult to obtain.

Your information is so obvious, yet so brilliant. I shall pray for your continued strength and courage in getting this message to all humanity. Sincerely, D. S., M.Sc., L.M.P.

Depression; Suicidal:

August 1995, I first became aware of your book: *Your Body's Many Cries for Water.* I will be forever grateful for your years of research in reference to the role of water in the functioning of the human body. The chapter in the book pertaining to depression was the solution to over ten years of struggle in my life.

In your book, your simple formula of drinking water at the rate of a minimum of two quarts (64 oz. = 8 glasses) per day plus salt of 1/2 teaspoon over a 24-hour period has been the answer for my depression. Because of my weight, I followed the additional suggested formula of 1/2 the body weight number = the ounces of water required to properly keep all the cells fully hydrated. I make sure that I ingest at least 1/2 a teaspoon of table salt (sodium chloride) with my food during the same 24-hour period.

I am a 68-year-old retired professional chemical engineer. I had battled depression symptoms from 1985 until 1995. My wife, a nurse clinician, passed away in 1984. I was forced into early retirement after 33 1/2 years with a major oil company in 1985. Those familiar with the role of high stress causing dehydration, as Figure 9 in your book, will understand my problem. In addition, I had bought into the idea that a low-salt diet was the way of good health. Thus all the factors were in place for my body to show symptoms of depression. What I now know is that most of the anti-depressants used to treat patients with depression are also diuretics. I always manifested the symptom of extreme dry mouth sensation after being placed on anti-depressants. The symptom of anxiety then comes forth because of the additional need for water by the body. Add a prescribed anti-anxiety pill and the patient (me) was on chemical teeter-totter trying to achieve a balance of a normal life. Plus, in the *Physicians Desk Reference (PDR)*, in the listing for the above medications is the nice word "suicide." I have struggled when on anti-depressants and anti-anxiety medication with the fleeting surges of the mind of wanting to die. However, I never had the courage to act out the desire. The ultimate solution that worked for me: Water and salt; the simple answer.

In summary, for over a year I have been free of the need to take any medication of any kind. In December 1995, I qualified with no medical restrictions for a Class physical for a private pilot's license. In addition, my annual eye check revealed that my eye peripheral vision had improved relative to previous annual tests. My belief is that the cells in the eye have become better hydrated and I can read now without glasses.

May the value of your research and protocol continue to spread and be understood.
Sincerely, C. D., BS Chemical Engineering

Note: C. D. is well and able to cope with the adversities of life. He lost his business and came through it without any repercussions on his health. He now lectures to the residents of old-age homes.

◊ ◊ ◊

Depression; Suicidal:

Thank you and thank God for you! Your book, *Your Body's Many Cries for Water*, has made a tremendous difference in my life.

I suffered from "clinical depression" for over 22 years. My journey through the medical madness began with a psychologist who treated me with hypnotism. Another one tried to talk "it" away. My psychiatrist treated me with a number of different medications, including Pamelor, lithium, Prozac, Paxil, Neurontin, Depakote, Wellbutrin and Effexor. None of these medications worked as well as your water Rx. I have been medication free for several months and the side effects are wonderful. I have a marked increase in energy, restful sleep (without nightmares), a clear drug-free head, softer skin and hair and a noticeable decrease in appetite. More importantly, I have a will to live. The medications only served to keep me from killing myself. And they didn't do that very well either. I was hospitalized once for four days (self-admit), because suicide was looking like a pretty good option.

I have told, and will continue to tell everyone, I can about your water Rx that not one more minute of time be wasted in needless physical or mental suffering. That not one more dollar be wasted and one more life be lost.
Sincerely, C. M. K.

Note: Lithium—used in some emotional problems—behaves as if it is a salt substitute. However, it is not as effective in all chemical actions as ordinary salt.

🌢 🌢 🌢

Depression:

I am writing to comment on and express my thanks for your research and your book *Your Body's Many Cries for Water.* I found it very concise and logical in its presentation and helpful in its message.

I would also like to relay my experience prior to reading your book and the implementation of drinking more water. I have no physical illness that I am aware of and enjoy good health, yet for all of my adult life I struggled with depressive states. These states are not predictable and I have found little effective remedy other than simply to endure and wait. Without describing my depression I can say that for me it was often near debilitating and I have as a consequence done considerable experimentation in an effort to find relief. I have tried numerous therapies, both additive and subtractive. In the additive, I've tried acupuncture, homeopathy, Chinese herbs, western herbs, chiropractic, sound and color therapy, chemical drugs, vitamins, essential oils, more light, colon cleansing, ozone and oxygen supplements, meditation, individual and group psychotherapy, macrobiotic diet and more exercise. In the subtractive I have eliminated amalgam fillings, caffeine, meat and sugar, alcohol and drugs, and all foods, during certain periods in my life. In regards to the effects of these trials I can say that only the increasing exposure to natural sunlight and use of anti-depressant chemical drugs have had a noticeable effect on my depression. I still get more sunlight but have abandoned drugs due to unacceptable side effects and concerns over long -term dependency.

I read *Your Body's Many Cries for Water* nearly three months ago and started drinking at least 8 glasses of water a day two months ago. I think that after this time I can with relative certainty say that there has been a marked improvement in my mood and absence of depressive states. This I say as a general statement. There are times when I feel low, but on the whole I feel much improved. I have much humor and my thoughts are much more optimistic. I have observed that even a single day without drinking water has a negative effect.

I feel compelled to thank you for your work and for bringing it to the public. Although I cannot comment on the relationship between drinking more water and other maladies, I would not hesitate to recommend the book and the practice of drinking more water to anyone who struggles with depression.
Cordially, J. W.

**Whiplash; Pain;
Depression:**

How many times do we need to hear the "stuff" before we get it. At the same time I am comforted knowing my Creator never gives up on me and the truth keep returning!

June 13 our car was rear-ended and both Jack and I were injured. Because I was turned twisted so to speak, watching for oncoming traffic, I received a whiplash to my hip. Did not feel hurt immediately however 3 days later I felt like I had been beaten! Went to the chiropractor and massage therapist and acupuncturist... and with their treatments got periodic relief from the pain and interestingly enough they would say, "drink water;"—however, I made no connection with pain and dehydration!

I have never taken so much arnica, even resorted to Advil; some days I resorted to ice pack/heating pads, to rochanteric belt, to lumbar support belt. Outcome: major depression. What is going to happen! Then an article appeared 10 days ago in a local paper about Dr. B's work written by a local massage therapist, about connection of pain and dehydration. I thought, I have nothing to lose.

Next morning upon arising I immediately drank about 32 ounces of water and then continued throughout the day to get in about 80

ounces. About 3 days later I began to sense the pain diminishing. All this time I have been having treatments with some improvement, but still the lingering pain. After 5 days on the water I had an almost pain-free day! Then on the 6th day pain free and have been since—truly it was the water—also lost a couple of pounds with no change to exercise or diet; and my energy returned. My depression lifted and I am back to my energetic loving self. So yes I am on a mission to spread the word. I am so glad you are doing such a fine job.
Love, Jeanne

♦   ♦   ♦

Chronic Fatigue; Depression:

Every day since I began your wonderful water & salt program, I read and reread your remarkable book *Your Body's Many Cries for Water* and continue to be impressed by the many ways in which your new paradigm brings to light the true etiology of the many diseases that are prevalent.

My excitement is mounting day-by-day, as I find my energy, clarity and sense of well-being improving.

After struggling with debilitating chronic fatigue syndrome and acute depression for almost ten years now, I am very grateful for your remarkable insight and for your persistence in bringing this information to the public and scientific community.

I will be ordering a case of your paperbacks to send to friends and relations who are suffering from misdiagnosed illnesses.

May you live a very long life so that your research can continue and so that your teachings can spread around the world.
With deep appreciation, D. G., Ph.D.

Heartburn; Asthma;
Depression; Allergies:

Until I read your book, *Your Body's Many Cries for Water*, I suffered from:

- Heartburn/hiatus hernia
- Asthma
- Various allergies
- Slowing down of memory
- Arthritis
- Depression

I seldom went out without a pocket of antacid tablets; I used them after every meal. I would have asthma attacks several times a week, usually when stressed and in cold weather.

My memory began to slow down. After teaching for over thirty years, not being able to recall information immediately not being able to remember names or where I had put my glasses, etc, left me angry, frustrated and distressed.

I had arthritic aches and pains in varying degrees for years, and found that Prozac really helped although it dried me out and made me sleepy.

As soon as I read your remarkable book I started on your daily water routine and was amazed at the results in just a couple of days. The heartburn was gone, I haven't taken an antacid tablet since—I doubt if I shall ever need them again!!!

The asthma attacks have gone too. My memory is definitely improving—dramatically!!

I haven't had any arthritic aches and pains either. I'm also taking a holiday from the Prozac.

I seldom drank just water alone. I drank some eight cups of tea a day, no soft drinks and almost no alcohol. Now I drink very little tea indeed. So, drinking some eight glasses of water a day was a big change in my liquid intake, but I feel great. I feel toned up and free, amazingly so, of the things that plagued me.

I am profoundly grateful for your book, your observations, your insights and learning and your generosity in taking time to speak with me and for the gift of improving incredibly my feeling of well being. I've been telling everybody I know about your book.
Yours sincerely, C. S.

Peptic Ulcer; Asthma:

I have been attempting to drink 6–8 glasses of water daily since receiving the *Last Chance Report* vol. 3, number 5, and am pleased to report remarkable results.

My peptic ulcer that has bothered me for years has gone into remission. I have been on anti-acid pills for years too and no longer need them routinely—just rarely use one. I no longer take Tagamet and medicines like that. For years I have had a habit of (addiction to) Cokes. I am happy to say that I immediately stopped craving for them after starting my water project. Also, my asthma has diminished noticeably. I am delighted with all the progress I have made just on water.

I am 65 and recently retired and really feeling very good and most certainly intend to continue drinking water as suggested. I am sure that there are many other benefits I am receiving from drinking water in quantities like I do now.

It hardly seems enough to just say thanks, but be sure that I am very, very grateful for this revelation.

Best wishes, G. W.

P.S. Of course I have known for years that I should be drinking more water, but thought it was too much trouble and was not motivated to do so until I got your report.

**Peptic Ulcer; Colitis Pain;
Hypertension:**

After reading your book *Your Body's Many Cries for Water*, I recognized my own problems were like those mentioned. I had stomach ulcer, colitis pain, high blood pressure that nothing seemed to help. After a short period of benefit from a blood pressure medicine, I had more side effects than help, so you can imagine how glad I was to read of your book reviewed in Sam Biser's *Health Newsletter*.

After only a few months, I'm not taking anything for any of these conditions except drinking at least 8 glasses of water a day, and feeling great! Thank you, M. H.

Peptic Ulcer:

I promised you over three years ago that I would write and tell you how the water worked for my ulcer. Great! Great! I really believe you saved my life. I had been hospitalized for ulcers four times; the last three, for bleeding ulcers. Then I read your book and talked to you twice on the phone. You assured me it would work, and it did. I haven't had any problem with my (40-year) ulcer in 3 years. I have sold over 200 copies of *Your Body's Many Cries for Water* in my health food store. I want to meet you sometime. Maybe there is something sometime I can do for you.
Sincerely yours, Dr. George C. Reed

Peptic Ulcer; Acid Reflux:

Since I was 18 years old, I have suffered from stomach and digestive problems. In the beginning, my doctor had me go for an ultra-sound of my stomach and gallbladder. The only thing they found were two ulcers, so I was given Zantacs and told the ulcers would heal in six weeks. For the next six years, I experienced severe stomachaches, heartburn and would often make myself sick just so the burning would go away. By the time I was 25, I could only eat baby food and ice cream. Every time I would try to eat, I would feel as though there was something stuck in my throat. I went to the emergency room; all they did was blood work, which cost me $400.00.

Next, I went to my medical doctor who told me it was my nerves and sent me home with Zantacs and BuSpar to help me relax. Now I was having anxiety attacks from not being able to eat, needless to say none of these pills helped me so I said I want to go to an ear/nose/throat specialist. When I went to him, he put the scope up my nose, down through as far as my voice box; he found nothing wrong, sent me home with nose sprays and pills, stating it must be allergies. By now my nerves were shot so I talked to my friend who is a chiropractor and began going to him for treatments of my neck and shoulders. My muscles were very tight and I had knots in the muscles on the side of my neck, which were causing severe spasms making me feel like someone was choking me.

By maintaining the amount of stress and going for treatments, I was feeling better but still had heartburn and, by nighttime, my throat was so dry that my voice was hoarse. I couldn't even read a book to my daughters. I spoke to my doctor about these problems and he suggested an upper GI series to see if I may have a hernia. Another $200.00 and all they found was that I had severe acid reflux, which they felt was caused from stress. My first thought were "here we go again, more tests, more money and no relief."

I explained to my chiropractor and he felt we should do a series of blood work and check my thyroid gland. Another $200.00 for blood work that came back showing my calcium was up and every thing else was normal except for my red blood cells, which were up. He said it wasn't a bad thing, just to drink more fluids. When my husband was telling Bob Butts about my medical problems, he gave him some tapes and papers on drinking water—"nature's cure"—for me to try. Well, to be honest, I didn't believe drinking water would help me eat and not get the fullness in my throat, but I can tell you it WORKS! I drink approx. 2 quarts of water a day, no soda, no tea, no coffee, and I am able to eat REAL FOOD these days, even cucumbers which I always loved but I was never able to eat because of the burning and heartburn after. I have not experienced a dry mouth, sore throat or much heartburn since.

About 30 days after starting the water program, I feel better today than I have felt in years. I eat right, drink my water, reduced stress and I am looking forward to enjoying a healthy life without digestive complaints.

Come to my 26th birthday party in July and we will all toast with a tall cold glass of ice water.
Sincerely, M. G.

＊   ＊   ＊

Allergies; Joint Pain;
Irritable Bowel; Angina:

Thanks very much for writing your great book *Your Body's Many Cries for Water*. I soaked up the info like a sponge. It was information that I had longed to hear all of my life, since I've had a problem ranging from allergies to triple bypass, joint pains, total hair loss, mitral valve ring emplacement, colon or irritable bowel syndrome. These are all cries of dehydration. Even with all those problems I always seem to survive. Just a few years back at the age of 56, a friend of mine and myself got into a battle to see who could lose the most weight. I lost the battle, but we both loved to ride bikes.

We started our own small 10-mile rides and after about six months we decided to ride from San Antonio, TX, to El Paso, which is 594 miles. We did it in seven days, averaging 85 miles a day. I had a heart attack 4 years prior to the ride, so the doctor had me taking Procardia for the heart, a calcium channel blocker and prednisone for asthma, that I had acquired because they also had previously given me Inderal. This caused me to have asthma. So I am being given these toxic chemicals and I knew deep down inside me that this was the wrong thing to do. In 1987 I had angina pains again. The doctor did another angioplasty. I continued to ride my bike but I didn't have the stamina that I had enjoyed in 1986. In 1990, I had another episode with angina and went back again for another angioplasty and was told to discontinue using

Procardia and they put me on a Cardizem, another calcium blocker. In 1991 I was under a lot of stress at work, but this time they said I didn't have any new blockage. In 1994 I was having water buildup and they put me in the hospital for CHF and I urinated 20 lbs of water. When I came out of the hospital I weighed 175 pounds. The doctor wanted to do a bypass on me and I said, "no way."

In 1996 I was really feeling angina pains and swelling with edema. I gave in to the bypass and a mitral valve ring. I have a new doctor. He had me on Cozaar for high BP and Lasix diuretic 80 mg twice a day, and potassium supplement, CoQ10 and a magnesium supplement and has tried to get me to take Lipitor and Zocor to lower my cholesterol. I refused to take the latter as I have read that it is known to deplete CoQ10. I asked him at one time if it would be advisable to drink more water and he said no. I have been lied to for years. I know that supplements are supposed to strengthen a weakened body, but I never gave them a chance since I didn't drink enough water. I didn't drink any more than 3 glasses of water a day. I drank a couple of glasses of wine and 16 oz. cans of beer because I liked their taste.

I have always consumed beer and wine; just this week I began drinking more water. I noticed my blood pressure dropped from 150/90 to 128/80. That encouraged me to know that the water was not going to build up in my lungs and ankles. I was amazed at my kidneys beginning to excrete the water normally. The strange part of this is that I didn't take Lasix or Cozaar for the entire week. I am ecstatic to say the least. I rode my bike six miles yesterday and today I started walking on my treadmill. I walked for 30 minutes. I also listen to a tape entitled *Perfect Health* by Dr. Paul Scheely of Learning Strategies Corporation. It's a great mental therapy for people who have been told their condition is irreversible. I believe the body can re-heal itself as you claim, with the proper diet and proper amount of plain water and a positive mental outlook. I am 71 years young and am now learning to play the guitar. Shame on me because I studied two years to be a chiropractor in 1954 but dropped out due to lack of insurance co. acceptance of chiropractic. I believe what you say is the truth and I believe your book should be next to the Bible. God Bless you!
Sincerely, C. E. W.

Alcohol; Pain;
Hypertension; Compacted Bowels;
Alligator Skin:

My life changed after two months on the "Water Cure." As the result of an accident on Oct. 5, 1954, I suffered a broken back, dislocated shoulder, dislocated knees, a smashed foot and a fractured skull. I've had severe pain and discomfort ever since. I was taking Lasix, a diuretic for edema of both legs. I also took Atenolol and Lisinopril for high blood pressure and was told to use no salt. I was a heavy consumer of alcohol most of my life. It got to where I was drinking one or two six-packs of beer each day and sometimes as much as a full case. I prayed to God to help me stop drinking.

I first heard about the "Water Cure" on *Positive Press on the Air*. My wife and daughter went to Cee-Kay Auto and spoke to Bob Butts about the "Water Cure." I sat in the car. It wasn't easy for me to come in. I read the literature and it made sense to me, so I tried the "Water Cure." The day I started drinking a gallon of water a day while using sea salt liberally, I quit drinking alcohol. I've had no desire for any since, even when in the company of others drinking alcohol. My pain is diminished to the point that I don't park in handicap spots. I am now off all pain medication. The edema in my ankles disappeared in two days. In two weeks my blood pressure returned to normal and I've been off the medication since. Before going on medication my pressure was 166 over 126. On medication it would be about 156 over 83. Now it is 141 over 78. My energy also greatly improved. It's incredible how much my life changed for the better in just two months.

I recommended the "Water Cure" to my daughter Kelly, who was suffering from compacted bowels. In five days she was restored to health. Her complexion also greatly improved. She had very severe blemishes and skin texture that was so bad it resembled alligator hide. It returned to almost normal in five days. She now feels like a million dollars. Feel free to share my success with your listeners and readers. You may use my name, address and telephone number.
Sincerely, M. K.

218

"The Moving Finger writes; and, having writ, Moves on: not all your Piety nor Wit Shall lure it back to cancel half a line, Nor all your Tears wash out a Word of it."

Omar Khayyam

The AMA and its members employed in medical teaching need to face the shocking reality that has now emerged:

The Washington Post
Wednesday, April 15, 1998

Correctly Prescribed Drugs Take Heavy Toll

Millions Affected By Toxic Reactions

By RICK WEISS
Washington Post Staff Writer

More than 2 million Americans become seriously ill every year because of toxic reactions to correctly prescribed medicines taken properly, and 106,000 die from those reactions, a new study concludes. That surprisingly high number makes drug side effects at least the sixth, and perhaps even the fourth, most common cause of death in this country.

Embarrassingly oblivious to the diverse ways in which chronic unintentional dehydration manifests in the human body, and having scuttled the introductory physiological and nutritional principles of earlier medical teachings in favor of the more lucrative chemical manipulation of dehydration-produced human health problems, physicians engaged in allopathic medicine have unwittingly permitted the drug industry to enroll them as their 007 agents, converting our once honorable healers' license into a license to kill. This shocking reality is background to the now correctable health-care crisis of all advanced societies in the twenty-first-century world.

God help humankind if the personal observations on the health benefits of water in this book do not stimulate readers to rise against the mainstream medical establishment, the government, and the Congress, and force them to take the side of the public against the medical fraud that is being practiced daily within the sick-care system in our country.

F. Batmanghelidj, M.D.

ABOUT THE AUTHOR

Dr. F. Batmanghelidj (pronounced Batman-ge-lij), American citizen, was born in Iran in 1931. He attended school in Scotland, and received his medical training at London University's St. Mary's Hospital Medical School. Upon completion of his studies, he had the privilege of being selected as a house doctor in his own medical school. Dr. Batmanghelidj practiced medicine in England before returning to Iran, where he helped develop hospitals and a family charity teaching medical center and sports center.

When revolution broke out in 1979, Dr. Batmanghelidj, as a member of a prominent family, was thrown in jail and was slated to be shot. While waiting to be "processed"as a political prisoner in Evin prison, he discovered the healing power of water.

One night, Dr. Batmanghelidj had to treat a fellow prisoner who was suffering severe peptic ulcer pain. With no conventional medication at his disposal, Dr. Batmanghelidj gave the man, who was crippled with pain, two glasses of water. Within eight minutes, his pain disappeared. He was instructed to drink two glasses of water every three hours, and he became absolutely pain-free for the four remaining months he was in prison. Without using any medication, he was cured. The dotor's discovery of the medicinal property of water at Evin also saved his own life. The authorities now wanted to be associated with his discovery.

During the thirty one months of his imprisonment, Dr. Batmanghelidj treated more than three thousand peptic ulcer sufferers with water alone. He conducted extensive research during his prison stay into the medicinal effects of water, and discovered water could prevent, relieve, and cure many painful, degenerative diseases. He found Evin prison an "ideal stress laboratory," and despite being offered an earlier release, he chose to stay an extra four months in prison to complete his research into the relationship of dehydration and bleeding peptic ulcer disease. A report of his findings was smuggled out of Iran and became the editorial article in the June 1983 issue of the *Journal of Clinical Gastroenterology*, which was reported on by the *New York Times* science section.

After his release from prison in 1982, Dr. Batmanghelidj escaped from Iran and came to America. He was instrumental in creation of the Foundation for the Simple in Medicine in 1983. He became engaged and directed the development of a molecular understanding of the effect of chronic unintentional dehydration on the human body. The foundation's findings were published in their *Journal of Science in Medicine Simplified* in 1991 and 1992 and are now posted on the Web site *www.watercure.com.*

His research at the foundation produced a paradigm shift in the basic science of medicine, when, as the guest lecturer of an international cancer conference, he explained that pain is a sign produced by dehydration in the human body. His paradigm shift article, "Pain: A Need for Paradigm Change," was published in the *Journal of Anticancer Research* in 1987. His studies show that, if we maintain a healthy lifestyle of drinking adequate water on a regular basis, we will be able to enjoy good health and avoid diseases and painful conditions that require pharmaceutical drugs and expensive medical procedures.

In 1989, at the 3rd Interscience World Conference on Inflammation, Dr. Batmanghelidj explained, for the first time in medical history, that histamine is a neurotransmitter in charge of water regulation and drought-management programs of the body—the medical breakthrough people have been waiting for.

Dr. Batmanghelidj now dedicates his time to promoting professional and public awareness of the healing power of water. His book, *Your Body's Many Cries for Water*, has helped millions of people live happier, healthier lives. He has been a guest on over two thousand radio talk shows and many television programs.

He has written five books in English: *Your Body's Many Cries for Water*, which has been translated into many languages; *How to Deal with Back Pain & Rheumatoid Joint Pain*; *ABC of Asthma, Allergies and Lupus*; *Water: For Health, For Healing, For Life* (published by Warner Books); and now, *Water Cures: Drugs Kill*. He has also written the Special Report on Arthritis and Back Pain. He has produced a ten-hour audiotape seminar, *Water, Rx for a Healthier, Pain-Free Life*, and four videotapes, *Cure Pain & Prevent Cancer; Dehydration & Cancer; Health Miracles in Water & Salt*; and the *Back Pain Video*. He has written a number of articles for health magazines. His most recent article, "Waiting to Get Thirsty Is to Die Prematurely and Painfully," is published in the *Townsend Letters for Doctors and Patients* in January 2003.

INDEX

INDEX

OTHER HEALTH EDUCATION PRODUCTS
By F. Batmanghelidj, M.D.

BOOKS

Your Body's Many Cries for Water, PB	$14.95
Your Body's Many Cries for Water, HC	$27.00
How to Deal with Back Pain & Rheumatoid Joint Pain	$14.95
ABC of Asthma, Allergies & Lupus	$17.00
Water: RX for a Healthier Pain-free Life	$7.00
Water for Health, for Healing, for Life	$14.95

VIDEOS

How to Deal with Back Pain	$29.95
Health Miracles in Water & Salt, Choice Medications For Cure of Pain and Disease, Including Cancer	30.00
Cure Pain & Prevent Cancer	$30.00
Dehydration and Cancer	$20.00

INDIVIDUAL AUDIO TAPES

Your Body's Many Cries for Water	$10.00
MS: Is "Water" its Cure?	$10.00
Water & Salt: RX for Total Healing	$10.00
Water: The New Immune Breakthrough & Pain and Cancer "Wonder Drug"	$10.00

AUDIO TAPE SERIES

Water: RX for a Healthier, Pain-Free Life

(Ten hours of in-depth information, 8 tapes) $67.00

Health Miracles in Water & Salt, Choice Medications

For Cure of Pain and Disease, Including Cancer (2 tapes) $18.00

CDs & DVD

The New Immune Breakthrough &

     Pain and Cancer "Wonder Drug" $18.00

Health Miracles in Water & Salt, Choice Medications

     For Cure of Pain and Disease, Including Cancer

     Set of 2 CDs $20.00

     DVD $30.00

For more information on the items above, see www.watercure.com.

Discounts available for 5 or more books

Shipping costs depend on weight.

For ordering and information concerning orders please contact:

e-mail: shipping@watercure.com

Phone: 1-800-759-3999 Monday - Friday, 9:00am to 5:00pm ET

Fax: 703-848-0028

Mailing address: Global Health Solutions

               8472A Tyco Rd.

               Vienna, VA 22182

Some scientific articles on molecular physiology/pathology of dehydration posted on the Website watercure.com

- A New and Natural Method of Treatment of Peptic Ulcer Disease

- Pain: A Need for Paradigm Change

- Neurotransmitter Histamine: An Alternative View Point -- Abstract of Presentation at the 3rd Inter-Science World Conference on Inflammation, etc.

- Receptor Down-Regulation

- Pain Signifies Thirst for Water

- AIDS - More Convincingly A Metabolic Disorder

- AIDS - Transglutaminase

- AIDS - The Dead End of Virus Etiology

- Tumor Necrosis Factor and HIV

- For The Record

- Science or Attitude

- Neurotransmitter Histamine

- Regulatory Role of Cellular Free Water

- Functions of Histamine and Gastroenterology

- Histamine and Serotonin: A Conceptual Approach to Carcinogenesis

- Paradigm Shift

- Tryptophan

- Water: A Pivotal Factor in Carcinoma of The Breast

Personal Notes:

Personal Notes:

Personal Notes:

Personal Notes: